An Introduction to
Research for Midwives

For my wife Brenda,
my sons Michael and David,
and my grandchildren Nia and Evan

Commissioning Editor: Mairi McCubbin
Development Editors: Helen Leng, Fiona Conn
Project Manager: Divya Krish
Designer/Design Direction: Charles Gray
Illustration Manager: Bruce Hogarth

An Introduction to
Research for Midwives

THIRD EDITION

Colin Rees BSc MSc PGCE
Lecturer, School of Nursing and Midwifery Studies, Cardiff University, Cardiff, Wales, UK

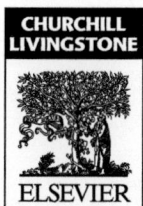

CHURCHILL LIVINGSTONE
ELSEVIER

© 2011 Elsevier Ltd. All rights reserved.

No part of this publication may be reproduced or transmitted in any form or by any means, electronic or mechanical, including photocopying, recording, or any information storage and retrieval system, without permission in writing from the publisher. Details on how to seek permission, further information about the Publisher's permissions policies and our arrangements with organizations such as the Copyright Clearance Center and the Copyright Licensing Agency, can be found at our website: www.elsevier.com/permissions.

This book and the individual contributions contained in it are protected under copyright by the Publisher (other than as may be noted herein).

First edition 1997
Second edition 2003
Third edition 2011

ISBN 978-0-7020-3490-9

British Library Cataloguing in Publication Data
A catalogue record for this book is available from the British Library

Library of Congress Cataloging in Publication Data
A catalog record for this book is available from the Library of Congress

Notices

Knowledge and best practice in this field are constantly changing. As new research and experience broaden our understanding, changes in research methods, professional practices, or medical treatment may become necessary.

Practitioners and researchers must always rely on their own experience and knowledge in evaluating and using any information, methods, compounds, or experiments described herein. In using such information or methods they should be mindful of their own safety and the safety of others, including parties for whom they have a professional responsibility.

With respect to any drug or pharmaceutical products identified, readers are advised to check the most current information provided (i) on procedures featured or (ii) by the manufacturer of each product to be administered, to verify the recommended dose or formula, the method and duration of administration, and contraindications. It is the responsibility of practitioners, relying on their own experience and knowledge of their patients, to make diagnoses, to determine dosages and the best treatment for each individual patient, and to take all appropriate safety precautions.

To the fullest extent of the law, neither the Publisher nor the authors, contributors, or editors, assume any liability for any injury and/or damage to persons or property as a matter of products liability, negligence or otherwise, or from any use or operation of any methods, products, instructions, or ideas contained in the material herein.

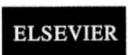

ELSEVIER — your source for books, journals and multimedia in the health sciences
www.elsevierhealth.com

Working together to grow libraries in developing countries
www.elsevier.com | www.bookaid.org | www.sabre.org

ELSEVIER | BOOK AID International | Sabre Foundation

The Publisher's policy is to use paper manufactured from sustainable forests

Printed and bound by CPI Group (UK) Ltd, Croydon, CR0 4YY
Transferred to digital print 2013

CONTENTS

Preface   vii

Acknowledgements   ix

1. Midwifery, research and evidence-based practice   1
2. Key concepts in research   17
3. The basic framework of research   31
4. Qualitative research approaches   43
5. Critiquing research articles   61
6. Reviewing the literature   77
7. The research question   91
8. Ethics and research   101
9. Surveys   117
10. Interviews   131
11. Observation   143
12. Experiments   155
13. Statistics in research   173
14. Sampling methods   197
15. The challenge of the future   215

Glossary of common research terms   227

Index   243

PREFACE

Since the publication of the second edition of this book, evidence-based practice has become one of the key features of healthcare in the UK and many other countries. Despite its apparent success, there is still a lack of clear understanding of what it is and how healthcare professionals can and should play their part in its use in clinical practice. It depends to a large extent on knowledge of research and the transfer of research findings into practice, following a careful evaluation of the quality of the research process that has produced it. This demands the use of skills and understanding and requires working together with other health professionals.

One of the main barriers to using research is 'the jargon', or worse, 'the statistics'. A further problem is that it is easy to forget some basic principles about research if you are not making frequent use of that knowledge. One solution to these problems is a simple book on research that will act as an effective resource: a friend who will inform, not intimidate. This is what you are holding in your hands.

The third edition of this book will help you demystify research and make the subject of research accessible whether you are a student or in clinical practice. It is written in a simple, practical and purposeful way to avoid reinforcing people's worst fears that research is simply unintelligible jargon. If you find any of the technical language confusing, there is an extensive glossary of terms at the back of the book where you will find clear explanations.

The book combines the following three themes:

1. Research methods and processes
2. The critical evaluation of research
3. The application of research to midwifery practice.

All the chapters in the third edition have had a thorough makeover: you will now find up-to-date references to research studies, the inclusion of new topic areas and extensively re-written chapters since the last edition.

Each chapter outlines a key research topic and explains major issues that need consideration before applying research to practice. The relationship between the midwife and research is examined from two perspectives: the midwife as the 'producer' of research, that is, carrying out research; the midwife as the 'user' of research, that is, critically assessing the research findings of others. Each role has different implications for the knowledge and skills required to achieve competence. These differences are clearly addressed at the end of each chapter under the heading 'Conducting research', which provides some practical advice on carrying out research, and 'Critiquing research', which outlines areas to consider when reading research reports. Each chapter ends with a list of key points that provide a summary of essential information.

Although textbooks are not meant to be read in a sequential order like a novel, Chapter 1 does set the scene by examining the relationship between the midwife, evidence-based practice, and research. Chapter 2 includes some fundamental concepts that will provide the groundwork for the remaining chapters, while Chapter 3 outlines the basic structure of research. Chapter 4 shows that research comes in a number of packages, and illustrates the relevance of qualitative research to midwifery. Once you have reached Chapter 5 (on critiquing), the order in which you read the other chapters becomes less important. Reading is a personal activity, however, and you may find a different route through the book. If it is used as part of a course, you may use it more like a reference book and dip in at strategic points when a session or assignment requires specific information. Whatever your reason for reading it, I hope you find it provides the answers to many of your questions about research and that it allows you to play an optimum role in evidence-based practice.

It is important to emphasise that this is an **introduction** to the extensive world of research. It is not meant to include chapters or sections on everything you may want to know on the subject. The topics that have been included are essential to an introduction to the subject. In particular, this book is built on the development of skills, not just the acquisition of knowledge. This approach has been used successfully over many years of teaching midwives, nurses and other health professionals. I hope you find it works for you.

Cardiff, 2010   Colin Rees

ACKNOWLEDGEMENTS

I would like to express my gratitude first and foremost to Fiona Conn, Helen Leng, and my project manager Divya Krish, at Elsevier, for their patience and wonderful support while I produced this third edition. It was not meant to take this long!

I owe a great deal to the support and friendship of many midwifery educationalists from my past who believed in my ability to enthuse their students with a passion for research. Illustrious people such as Sandy Kirkman and Gail Williams in Cardiff, and Christine Tucker and Sheena Payne at the University of the West of England in Bristol played a great part in allowing me to educate their students.

I would like to say a big 'thank you' to all the midwifery, nursing and other students who bought the previous editions of the book, especially those I have had the pleasure to teach, not only in the UK but also my students in Germany and Oman, as well as those working in the clinical setting for whom this book is especially written.

I would like to thank a special bunch of friends and work colleagues who have always supported me throughout my career. Thanks to Ian Hulatt, friend and best man, George McWhirter, for reading and making suggestions on the chapter on statistics in the second edition which has been included here, and a special thanks to Jerry Bray, who always enthusiastically supports my work and has been a great colleague and teaching partner in Oman. I would also like to thank my longstanding friend Andy Mardell, who provided practical support in helping me develop my research writing skills. I would also like to thank Sue Ward who has been a wonderful and cheerful office mate who makes a big difference to my working day.

For many years, I have also had tireless support and encouragement in my work and in the writing of this third edition from Dr Dianne Watkins who has always promoted my contribution to teaching. I would especially like to acknowledge her friendship, guidance and belief in me. I am also lucky enough to have Sheila Hunt as my Dean, who has similarly had faith in my teaching ability and supported my continued development within the School of Nursing and Midwifery Studies in Cardiff University. I have always admired her midwifery research and continue to include it in this edition as an example of how research in midwifery should be conducted.

In producing this edition, as with previous editions, I have received so much practical and emotional support from my wife, Brenda Rees, who has achieved so much and has inspired so many in her outstanding career in midwifery and women's health. Her encouragement, enthusiasm and care continue to make a huge difference to my life. I have so much to thank her for and greatly appreciate everything she has done for me.

In writing this third edition I have tried to include all the best aspects of the previous editions and make it fresh and relevant to the current context of health care. I believe research literacy is a crucial aspect of professional development and hope this book helps you in making your personal contribution to your profession. Thank you.

Midwifery, research and evidence-based practice

The principle philosophy of health care in the UK, as with other major countries in the world, is evidence-based practice. In midwifery, this means a focus on clinical outcomes for women and their babies that are based on clear evidence of their effectiveness. Although this philosophy is well-matched with the philosophy of midwifery, it does demand increasing skills of the midwife. These include information searching, gathering and synthesising skills, and those of critical analysis. In particular, it is important that midwives, in common with other health practitioners, are research literate, that is, they have an understanding of the principles of research and how it can be evaluated. For some, it also means contributing to the generation of knowledge through research activity. This first chapter prepares the way for the remainder of the book by exploring the context of research in modern midwifery and identifies some essential skills for the individual midwife.

Although this is a book on research, we cannot start without firstly discussing evidence-based practice. This is because the goals and expectations of health care from a national right down to an individual level are shaped by the demands of evidence-based practice. Clearly this is a powerful concept that every health professional needs to understand, as it dominates so much of the thinking in health care. Its relevance to midwifery has been emphasised by Cluett (2005) who believes evidence-based practice is the linchpin to contemporary woman–centred maternity care. This first chapter, then, traces the development and meaning of evidence-based practice and its implications for an understanding of research within midwifery.

THREE MAIN PLAYERS

Published research is now a necessary and frequently accessed source of midwifery knowledge. This means that midwives need to be involved in carrying out research and know how to make use of research in their clinical practice. These two themes covering the production and use of research lie within the context of evidence-based maternity services and influence the structure of this book. For this reason, we now examine the relationship between the three main players of firstly midwifery, research and evidenced-based practice so that we can see the relationship between them.

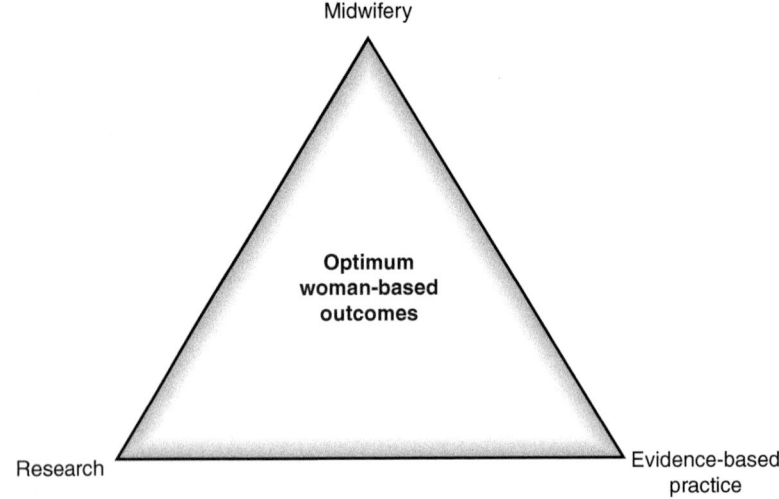

FIG 1.1 Providing optimum woman-based outcomes.

Figure 1.1 demonstrates the interrelationship that exists between midwifery, evidence-based practice and research. Starting at the top of the triangle, we can argue that the goal of midwifery is to provide support and care to women and their families to ensure best outcomes; whether these are physical, emotional or social. In addition, the key principle in achieving this goal is that care should be woman-centred. The relationship between a mother and midwife can take many forms, as indicated in the following statement from The International Confederation of Midwives (2005):

> *The midwife is recognized as a responsible and accountable professional who works in partnership with women to give the necessary support, care, and advice during pregnancy, labour, and the postpartum period, to conduct births on the midwife's own responsibility, and to provide care for the newborn and the infant. This care includes preventative measures, the promotion of normal birth, the detection of complications in mother and child, the accessing of medical care or other appropriate assistance, and the carrying out of emergency measures.*
>
> *The midwife has an important task in health counselling and education, not only for the woman, but also within the family and the community. This work should involve antenatal education and preparation for parenthood and may extend to women's health, sexual or reproductive health, and child care.*
>
> *A midwife may practice in any setting including the home, community, hospitals, clinics, or health units.*
>
> Adopted by the International Confederation of Midwives Council meeting, 19th July, 2005, Brisbane, Australia.

This is a complex and extensive remit. To achieve a high standard of care throughout these activities and settings, clinical decisions must be based on the best available information. This is the role of evidence-based practice, which forms the next point at the base of the triangle. The term *evidence-based practice* is defined in this book as:

> A problem-solving and decision-making system, based on the collection, evaluation and synthesis of sound evidence will ensure best practice by health professionals. This process should always be combined with professional judgement and the individual needs and desires of those receiving services.

The dominance of evidence-based practice in health care has led to it being seen as a 'movement' that has swept through so many countries and adopted as the preferred way of decision-making. This is illustrated in health policies and the activities of health organisations. A further definition of the process has been provided by Cleary-Holdforth and Leufer (2009: 286) as follows:

> Evidence-based practice is an holistic approach to care delivery that places the individual patient at its core. It is far more than research utilisation alone and is a partnership between interprofessional clinicians, patients and the best available evidence to optimise patient outcomes

Although this definition talks about 'patient' rather than 'woman' it can easily be transferred to midwifery with its emphasis on a holistic approach to support each woman.

The whole system of basing care on evidence has been made easier through the improved availability and accessibility of research carried out in health care. This has created an increase in midwifery knowledge based on research carried out by midwives, obstetricians and social scientists. The result has the potential to create high standards of decision making in maternity care. The philosophy and practice of evidence-based practice provides the energy that encourages the use of research knowledge and unites the two corners at the base of the triangle in Figure 1.1 above.

The far corner of the triangle underpinning both midwifery, and evidence-based practice is *research*. We can define research as:

> The systematic collection of information using carefully designed and controlled methods that answer a specific question objectively and as accurately as possible.

The result should be knowledge that increases our understanding of a topic or problem and which can be checked for accuracy. We should be able to apply this knowledge to a range of settings, not simply the one in which a study took place. In other words, research should be *generalisable*. This is one way in which quantitative research is judged: it should be capable of producing results that can be applied more generally (Polit and Beck 2008).

Evidence-based practice and research are not the same and should not be confused. Evidence-based practice focuses on the use or application of knowledge, usually that produced by research, in order to produce the highest standard of care and clinical outcomes. Research, on the other hand, is concerned with the production of knowledge that is as objective and accurate as possible. Evidence-based practice is the application of this knowledge as the foundation for clinical decision making. In this way, they can be seen as two distinct but related ingredients involved in the same process of improving midwifery care.

In summary, at the top of the triangle in Figure 1.1, evidence-based practice and research are used as tools as part of the practice of midwifery, to form the optimum clinical and care outcomes for a women and her baby, which forms the centre of the triangle. This model serves as a way of joining these different ideas in such a way that whichever point we choose to enter the model we can make sense of the way in which they are joined together and can see the bigger picture it represents.

WHY EVIDENCE-BASED PRACTICE?

We can argue the compatibility of evidence-based practice and midwifery with the following passage from Leufer and Cleary-Holdforth (2009):

> *EBP [evidence-based practice] is highly relevant in a social and healthcare environment that has to deal with consumerism, budget cuts, accountability, rapidly advancing technology, demands for ever-increasing knowledge and litigation* (p. 35).

This identifies many of the issues that confront midwifery care today and so provides motivation to embrace evidence-based practice as an integral part of maternity care. This point was made some time ago by Albers (2001) who was clear that the promotion of evidence-based care was consistent with the midwifery profession's core value of woman-centred care. This means that although relatively new, evidence-based practice is not an additional or peripheral aspect of midwifery care but is part of providing care in the same way as it is accepted in nursing and other professional groups in health care.

In addition, using evidence for clinical decision making is part of an ethical obligation for all health professionals, as it demonstrates the responsibility to 'do good' as a result of professional action and 'avoids doing harm'. In the language of ethical thinking, these are known as the obligations of *beneficence* (that is, doing good), and *non-maleficence* (that is, avoiding harm). This is supported by Roughley (2007) who suggests it is difficult to argue that midwives are in a position to guide women in decision making unless they have knowledge of the research that will enable women to make sound choices throughout pregnancy and the birth of their children. The professional duty to have up-to-date clinical knowledge is also reinforced through the following section in The Code (NMC 2008: 4):

- *You must deliver care based on the best available evidence or best practice.*
- *You must ensure any advice you give is evidence based if you are suggesting healthcare products or services.*

There are sound reasons, then, why midwifery has adopted the approach of evidence-based practice and all midwives are charged with supporting it. In the next section we will briefly consider the historical development of evidence-based practice so we can answer the question *'how did we get here?'*

THE RISE OF EVIDENCE-BASED PRACTICE IN HEALTH CARE

Within an incredibly short time period, evidence-based practice has become a global phenomenon, and is at the forefront of practice and health care provision in the UK (Dale 2005). According to Cullum et al. (2008), the term was first used in a publication in 1992 by Gordon Guyatt and the Evidence-Based Medicine Working Group where it was originally developed within the medical profession. It was introduced as a way of encouraging doctors to make use of the increasing amount of knowledge available through medical research to improve the standard of medical care. It was designed to replace tradition, intuition, or person preferences as the basis for decisions on patient investigations and treatments. The emphasis was on the '*science*' of medicine rather than the '*art*' of medicine.

The evidence-based movement spread rapidly from medicine to other health care groups including midwifery as an essential method of clinical decision making. Support for the approach swept through health policy and was the key message in the government report 'The New NHS: Modern, Dependable' (Department of Health 1997). The term 'evidence-based practice' is now common outside health care to include social work and areas such as evidence-based librarianship. This has led to it being promoted as a philosophy or way of thinking about professional decision making.

From recent beginnings, then, evidence-based practice has become a 'taken-for-granted' way of thinking about midwifery activity and in 2004 was said to be one of the most fashionable terms in health care (Rycroft-Malone et al. 2004). Despite this, the concept has been criticised on the grounds that it reduced the clinical freedom of practitioners to make their own decisions based on individual need and that it appeared to dismiss the experience of individual practitioners. In contrast, its supporters have argued there should be consistency and consensus in the way we carry out important clinical activities and these should reflect 'best practice', not the individual whims or preferences of the health professional. It has been argued that professional decisions should be influenced by objective or 'scientific' evidence that can be supported by well-conducted studies. This is because the evidence can be verified and demonstrated to be accurate. It is this aspect of being open to scrutiny by others and its accuracy tested that is not possible with individual experiences or opinions.

One implication of this move from experience to objective evidence has been that the 'expert' in the clinical area has moved from being someone with long or varied clinical experience, to someone who can find, evaluate and apply research findings to practice, and can integrate clinical standards or protocols into their own activities. This is a developing skill, as evidence is always changing and updating so protocols and guidelines need constant readjustment in line with latest evidence.

DEVELOPMENTS WITHIN MIDWIFERY

Midwifery has long made use of best practice guidelines and has established midwifery research links to prestigious multidisciplinary research units. One notable example has been the work of midwifery researches within the National Perinatal Epidemiology Unit (NPEU) Oxford, in the UK.

This research unit had been established by Ian Chalmers in 1978 with funding from the World Health Organization and the Department of Health, and consisted of a team of obstetric and midwifery researchers along with epidemiologists. Its work has included large research projects often with health policy implications, such as the Birthplace project, which was an integrated programme of research designed to compare clinical outcomes of 60 000 births planned in different settings such as home, different types of midwifery units, and in hospital obstetric units in England.

It was this unit that produced one of the early sources of midwifery evidence in the form of *A Guide to Effective Care in Pregnancy and Childbirth* (Enkin et al. 1989). According to Walsh (2010), the publication of this comprehensive summary of evidence allowed maternity care to move ahead of the game through the use of these guidelines based on randomised control trials. This was a paperback summary (without the references) of the two-volume, fully referenced version of *Effective Care in Pregnancy and Childbirth* (Chalmers et al. 1989) produced by the same team at the NPEU. The impetus to produce such a book had come following criticism from the influential British epidemiologist Archie Cochrane who had given obstetricians in the UK the 'wooden spoon' (loser's prize) in 1979 for the clinical speciality that made the least use of available research evidence (King 2005). As a result of this, Chalmers, along with other members from the NPEU, took up the challenge by producing a guide to best practice in obstetric care.

The historical significance of this book is that it was the forerunner of the electronic journal *The Cochrane Pregnancy and Childbirth Database of Systematic Reviews* in 1995. This later became *The Cochrane Collaboration* responsible for systematic reviews in all clinical areas, not just obstetrics, and has become respected throughout the world (available on-line at http://www.cochrane.org).

The availability of such resources, however, does not mean they will be used, as early work in midwifery by Stewart (2001) found. She explored what evidence-based practice meant to those within maternity services and discovered that at that time it was possible for strong evidence to exist but to be ignored by individuals who may select weaker or inappropriate evidence that supported personal beliefs, and reject or deny the evidence that did not support those beliefs. This ability of individuals to work within their own selective knowledge-base has been progressively replaced by a more consensual approach to ways of working. It is more usual now for standards of practice to be agreed in clinical areas and national guidelines produced by such powerful bodies as NICE (National Institute for Health and Clinical Excellence) adopted to inform practice. The use of guidelines and standards are then audited to ensure high levels of compliance. In this way there is now a greater consistency in approaches to clinical decision making to the benefit of those in contact with health services.

For many years, an important contributor to the midwifery knowledge-base has been the journal MIDIRS (*Midwives Information and Resource Service*). This provides access to a wide range of information on pregnancy, childbirth and infancy to assist in the improvement of maternity care through its journal and website (http://www.midirs.org/digest). Many student midwives and practising midwives have used its database to help locate relevant information.

It is resources such as this that have helped midwifery take an informed as well as challenging approach to much of the research that relates to maternity services and which acts as a basis for decision making.

Although there have been vast improvements in care as a result of evidence-based practice, it has to be recognised that further effort is needed. As some writers have suggested, gaps in research coupled with a lack of application of available research can still result in variations in practice (Roughley 2007). Although the introduction of evidence-based practice midwifery was seen as a powerful tool to question and examine obstetric-led decision making in maternity services (Munro and Spiby 2010), there has been a slow change away from some midwifery activities based on rituals and routines, and elements of continued support for decision making led by obstetricians. Research by Bluff and Holloway (2008), for instance, suggested that midwives as role models for student nurses could be divided into those that rigidly followed rules, often laid down by obstetricians, and those that were more flexible and woman centred rather than organisation centred. In other words, evidence-based practice was adopted to a variety of extents and perhaps not always with the intended consequences.

This problem of accepting the true spirit of evidence-based practice and achieving change is not unique to midwifery, but is a continuing threat to standards of care throughout health services. Improvements can be made through a clear understanding of evidence-based practice and its implications. The advantages of embracing evidence-based practice has been summed up by Cluett (2005:39) who asserts that *'the EBP midwife is a thinking, questioning, learning practitioner open to new ideas and ways of working'*. In other words, the future of the profession depends on those who can take it further and who are equipped with the skills of developing sound methods of working that produce the best results in the best way.

THE EVIDENCE-BASED PRACTICE PROCESS

Evidence-based practice comprises a number of clear steps identified by several authors (Sackett et al. 2000, Fineout-Overholt et al, 2005, Flemming 2008, Gerrish 2010). These are outlined in Figure 1.2.

The starting point is to identify an area for clinical improvement and develop a question that might guide the development of best practice. This question is frequently formed using the acronym PICO, which stands for **P**opulation-**I**ntervention-**C**omparison-**O**utcome. This was originally developed by Sackett et al. (1997), but is now used in this format or with slight variations by other writers (Craig 2007, Flemming 2008). So an example of PICO would be:

> In women during pregnancy (**P**) does attendance at antenatal groups (**I**), compared to those who do not attend groups (**C**), result in a higher level of women choosing to breastfeed their baby (**O**)?

The most important aspect of this kind of statement is that the 'outcome' must be measurable. So, statements such as is it 'better' or 'more effective' for women to attend antenatal groups are difficult to answer as there is no indication of how we would measure either outcome statement. In comparison, breastfeeding rate is measureable.

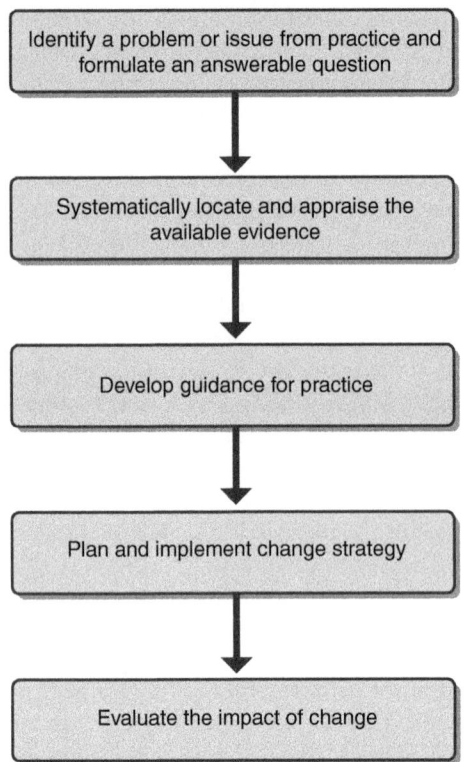

FIG 1.2 The process of evidence-based practice. (Based on Gerrish 2010)

The various elements of the PICO statement, then, guide the search for relevant literature through the use of each key word in the PICO question. The appropriate literature is systematically examined to provide a sound answer to that question. However, the literature should only be included if it has been critically evaluated and reaches a high standard. If the result is seen as strong or 'robust' enough to be used in practice, guidelines are drawn up and implemented. After a sufficient period of time the results of applying the new practice are evaluated to ensure that it should continue to be used and can be demonstrated to have had an impact on the outcome measure.

Although this is a very simplified model of the process, it does highlight some of the skills required by the midwife, such as the ability to carry out a comprehensive review of literature that includes high-quality articles capable of providing sound evidence. Midwives also need critiquing skills that will allow them to assess how well research has been carried out. A decision then has to be made on whether the evidence collected is adequate or sufficient to solve the problem in the particular local clinical area so that the decision to apply the findings can be made. Finally, there is a need to know how to evaluate clinical outcomes and ensure that they have the desired effect.

This is a considerable demand on the individual midwife. However, it is not envisaged that all midwives should be carrying out all these stages in relation to every one of their clinical activities. This is clearly not possible.

It is something that should be the responsibility all those involved in a clinical area or geographical area bound by the same systems. In other words, the agreeing of standards or guidelines for practice should be a team effort and can be based on nationally available guidelines or those developed locally. An illustration of this is Spiby and Munro's (2007) work on guidelines to support midwifery-led care in labour.

A possible misunderstanding from Figure 1.2 is that clinical decisions should be made solely on the basis of the literature. This, too, cannot be the case, as evidence, particularly in the form of research evidence, is not always available, or may be weak research that should not be used as the basis for decision making. A number of writers have been clear that decisions should not be made on the literature alone but as part of a combination of the literature, the individual (or group) clinician's expertise, and the values and preferences of those receiving care (Burns and Grove 2009: 11). In other words it is a synthesis between the three aspects of:

1. evidence,
2. professional knowledge and experience,
3. the expressed needs and views of those concerned.

Cullum et al. (2008: 2) support this by saying that *'research findings alone do not dictate our clinical behaviour'* but they should be used in combination with other considerations in the process of clinical decision making. In midwifery, the principle of *'woman-centred care'* (Leap 2009) fits comfortably into this evidence-based framework as it values a woman's individual needs rather than those of the health care organisation, whilst still providing the best level of clinical care amongst alternative options.

Evidence-based practice, then, is a clear step-by-step activity that seeks to provide the best clinical decisions. It is a logical process that requires skill in those applying it. In most situations, the guide to practice, the result of this process, will already exist and have been agreed by clinical areas. The individual practitioner must be satisfied that these have been based on carefully evaluated information and that they are up to date. If that is confirmed, then such guidelines have the potential to increase the quality of care available, and should form part of the decision-making process for the individual midwife.

RESEARCH AS EVIDENCE

One of the most frequently asked questions about evidence-based practice, according to Rycroft-Malone et al. (2004), is *'what counts as evidence'*. This is because there can be many sources of information used by clinicians on a daily basis, all of them potentially legitimate sources of evidence. The answer for medicine, the originator of this approach, was that research findings, particularly randomised control trials, were the main form of evidence. However, other groups, including midwives, have argued that there should be a broader definition of what counts as legitimate evidence. For example, Walsh (2008) includes qualitative research, intuition and ancient wisdom in what he sees as sources of evidence. You might like to think about what might be both the advantages and disadvantages of these examples.

It is clear, looking at those countries supporting evidence-based practice, that research remains the main source of evidence. Indeed, Polit and Beck (2008: 31) say that there is general agreement that rigorous research is paramount when it comes to deciding what counts as evidence. Why is this? Firstly, research provides a fit between the type of evidence it produces and the decisions that have to be made in health care. In other words, it seems to be 'fit for purpose' and relevant. To be relevant, Burns and Grove (2009: 12) suggest that:

> '... research evidence must focus on the description, explanation, prediction, and control of phenomena important to practice'.

This is exactly what midwifery research provides, and throughout this book practical examples will be given that cover these broad areas of importance to clinical decision making.

A further reason for the emphasis on research is that for evidence to be credible it has to come with some kind of safeguard on its accuracy, and it must be capable of being transferred to a variety of appropriate clinical settings. This means that audit or personal experience may be untypical and difficult to generalise to other situations. They possess little in the way of convincing argument on their accuracy or generalisability. Similarly, there is little to demonstrate that personal experience has been objectively gathered and verified.

Are all methods of collecting research evidence equally up to standard? This is important as not all methods of collecting information are equally convincing or accurate. Because of this, early supporters of evidence-based practice proposed that there should be a 'hierarchy' of evidence that would remind users that different forms of evidence should have a different weight attached to them, depending on the extent to which they demonstrate the elements that made them trustworthy or fit the criteria of sound evidence. At the top of the hierarchy were systematic literature reviews of randomised control trials. A systematic review is a very careful assessment of only high-quality research and, where possible, the findings of such research are combined together to overcome the difficulties found in individual research studies, such as a small sample size. Interestingly, this approach to comparing and synthesising high-quality research studies was exactly what Archie Cochrane had promoted so many years ago and which led to the Cochrane database.

Systematic reviews of the literature are followed in such hierarchies of evidence by high-quality single randomised control trials that clearly demonstrated the qualities of well-produced research. Further down the hierarchy were less 'scientific' forms of research including qualitative studies ending with alternatives such as professional opinion or experience. Again, there has been much opposition to such hierarchies in both nursing and midwifery where it has been argued that the emphasis on clinical trials and measurable outcomes are not the only relevant factors in care, but that experience, including that found in qualitative methods, is just as important.

Although qualitative studies are ranked toward the bottom of many of the hierarchies of evidence, it is important to say that this is because of the context in which discussions on research took place, and this was frequently in regard to questions of measurement and researcher objectivity in the research process.

As we shall see in Chapter 4, qualitative research does follow clearly defendable processes to support the truthfulness of findings, although the ability to generalise the findings are not comparable to other research situations. Nevertheless, such studies have a special role to play in midwifery research because of the concern not only with clinical outcomes but also with the quality of the journey through pregnancy and birth, where there are other criteria than simply measurable outcomes. For example, the experiences of home birth, birthing twins, or having a premature infant in a neonatal unit are all topics that can inform 'best practice'. For these kinds of life events, qualitative data is more appropriate and can inform both midwifery practice and policy. However, such research still needs to be rigorously conducted and so meet the criteria of sound evidence. This book will help you develop your understanding and skills to consider this type of qualitative evidence developed from the social sciences rather than the medical sciences. Midwifery, like nursing, is concerned with a wider scope and interpretation of science relevant to professional practice and so the interpretation of 'evidence' will be somewhat different from traditional medical thinking when it comes to what is judged as 'fit for purpose'.

COMPARISON BETWEEN SOURCES OF EVIDENCE

One way to understand the emphasis on research as a major source of evidence is to compare it against alternative forms of decision making, such as those suggested by Polit and Beck (2008: 12–13). The list below (Table 1.1) includes some of the major alternatives to research that have influenced decision making and provides an opportunity to consider some of the advantages and disadvantages of each source against those of research.

This is a varied list and, although each of these has its advantages, we can see that they all have a number of disadvantages that limit their accuracy and transferability to other clinical situations. Interestingly, although clinical experience has historically been accepted as a strong basis for decision making, Walsh (2008) presents some clear examples to suggest that clinical experience can lead to poor decision making. He includes such dangers as 'overconfidence' when predicting the way clinical events will unfold. Clinical predictions are well known for turning out to be wrong, and Walsh (2008) comments that studies have demonstrated that clinical predictions are often wildly inaccurate. He also refers to 'base-rate neglect' where clinicians can overestimate the prevalence or risk of something developing that is far from the actual level or frequency. Having a long clinical experience or being in a senior position, then, does not necessarily result in a superior source of evidence. In this situation, well-conducted research is more valuable compared to other forms of decision making because, in the words of Polit and Beck (2008: 13):

> Research conducted within a disciplined format is the most sophisticated method of acquiring knowledge that humans have developed.

Its main assets include the careful and closely controlled approaches to gathering evidence and the scrutiny it undergoes to ensure its accuracy. Although we should not have complete faith in every single study, the way research is presented allows us to inspect how the information was collected

AN INTRODUCTION TO RESEARCH FOR MIDWIVES

Table 1.1 Advantages and disadvantages of different sources for decision making

Source of decision making	Advantages	Disadvantages
Tradition	Familiar and accepted source of making decisions, especially by those receiving care and interventions. Little thought required on best clinical approach (do as we have always done).	May have been superseded by more effective methods. Clinical solutions may not have kept pace with changing demands and circumstances. Solutions can be quite narrow, and do not suggest adequate thought is given to personal circumstances or alternative more effective options. The basis for traditional approaches may have not been open to scrutiny and verification. Are there tested grounds to believe them? N.B. this method is not in line with current thinking within health care that demands decisions based on convincing evidence.
Authority	Accepted as strong guide to knowledge and decision making.	Decisions are made by those with the power to influence procedures and practices. May not be based on evidence. May be outdated.
Clinical experience	If a solution worked before it may work again. Taken as a strong source of knowledge in the past where experience was seen as providing 'wisdom'.	Experience may be untypical or results may have been 'one-off' outcomes, may not work again. A number of biases associated with professional experience and expertise have also been noted (Walsh 2008).
Trial and error	Appears systematic approach, has pseudo-scientific air of comparing approaches until a solution is found.	May stop at a workable solution although better solution may not have been reached. Not a very professional approach to care.
Intuition	Sometimes seems uncannily accurate. Provides a starting point for action.	May be drawing on subconscious memory of legitimate information and not a sudden or spontaneous source of knowledge. Not a professional basis for decision making. Difficult to teach new or student practitioners.
Logical reasoning	Has potential to arrive at a correct decision. Provides rational case for action.	May be flawed logic. Depends on accuracy of information used and powers of logic.
Assembled information (already existing data such as Caesarean section or infection rates, etc.)	Can provide a useful indication of trends or outcomes. Appears evidence-based.	Depends on accuracy of the data gathered, the method used to gather the data and the age of the data. Findings in one area may not be transferable to other area.
Research	Highly regarded as a source of knowledge. Well-conducted research reduces personal bias and controls for other influences and explanations. High level of transferability.	Can be poorly conducted. Too high a level of control of other influencing factors in the study setting might reduce the transferability of the information to other situations. May be inbuilt biases in situations. Can be overwhelming 'threats' to validity where results can be explained by other factors.

from participation in research. They point out that in the past members of vulnerable groups were overrepresented in potentially risky research and underrepresented in potentially beneficial research. Justice, then, related to fair play in who is involved in studies and the way in which potential benefits are distributed amongst those taking part.

PROBLEMS IN RESEARCH

The application of principles to practice is never easy, and ethical dilemmas are common in research. One example is that of informed consent. Part of respecting the individual is to ensure that the purpose of the research is made clear so that the individual is in a position to truly give informed consent. However, there are occasions where it is difficult to give comprehensive details of the study without compromising the validity of the results. There are situations where revealing the purpose of the study will influence the expectations or behaviour of the participants. For example, a study of student midwives' hand-washing techniques may not be accurate if the students are told that the thoroughness of their hand-washing technique is being observed. To gain more valid results, the researcher may have to say that they are observing routine procedures, and not draw attention to the importance of hand washing. The argument for this kind of incomplete disclosure would have to be made in the application to the LREC.

Another problem area for the researcher is that of confidentiality. We tend to think of confidentiality as not sharing information. Clearly, the purpose of research is to communicate and publish the results, but in a way that will not identify or harm the individual participant. However, at the point of data collection there are instances where it is not possible to keep confidences, even where this may be expected. One example is where there is a greater obligation on the midwife researcher to inform others of information that has been given in confidence. Clearly, where a respondent in an interview provides evidence physical abuse by a partner to them or their children, the midwife researcher would have to state that the information could not be kept confidential. The first course of action would be to encourage the respondent to report the matter, or to give permission for the researcher to report it. If this option was declined, the midwife researcher would have to report the information. The same would apply to interviews, or observation of staff involving unsafe or unethical practices. The researcher would have to intervene in the activity and report the matter. To overcome any problems in relation to confidentiality, a researcher must be clear in explaining the exact limits of confidentiality during the study. Similarly, if in interviews the respondent uses phrases such as 'between ourselves' or 'I shouldn't be telling you this but', the researcher should caution the individual that certain information would have to be reported.

CONDUCTING RESEARCH

This chapter has identified the main areas to consider when planning research. All NHS research in the UK must conform to agreed standards as set out in the clinical governance framework (DoH 2005) or, if the research is sponsored social research, the Framework for Research Ethics (ESRC 2010), and it is right and proper that it does. The most important principles to address are those of:

- informed consent,
- assessment of risks/benefits,
- confidentiality of material and anonymity of participants,
- fair selection and treatment of subjects.

At the planning stage it is important to determine the whole processes involved in carrying out research according to research governance, and how research approval is conducted in your clinical area or organisation. This can be quite a long chain of events, part of which will be approval by an LREC. The necessary forms for approval are available on line and advice on the procedure can be gained from the National Research Ethics Service (NRES) at http://www.nres.npsa.nhs.uk/applications/apply/ethical-review-requirements.

A great deal of thought needs to go into completing the forms for ethical approval, so you will find the RCN guidelines on Research Ethics (RCN 2007) useful in ensuring that you illustrate that ethical principles have been identified and addressed in the design of the study.

In research proposals, it must be clear that written informed consent will be gained, and that details of the study will be given in writing to those taking part. This will include a clear statement that there is no requirement to participate in the study, and that an agreement to take part is made on a voluntary basis. It should also be clear that the individual can withdraw at any point without this affecting care. Both the consent form and study information sheet should be written in plain language and included with the proposal to the LREC.

The submission to the ethics committee should demonstrate the major benefit of conducting the study and illustrate how the findings would make a contribution to practice. Careful use of the available literature and details of the local situation should be used to support these claims.

Where the applicant is new to research, it is expected that a supervisor with research experience will be named. This might be someone within midwifery education, or someone with previous research experience. Similarly, where the study will entail statistical analysis, the names of those providing statistical advice and support will be required to provide assurance on the accuracy of the results. Details on how confidentiality and anonymity will be maintained should be included. If names of subjects are not required, do not ask for them. Information on the arrangements for secure data storage should be outlined. Finally, it is important to assure the ethics committee that the researcher will not raise expectations that the study will result in the provision of additional services or facilities for those who take part.

Before submitting a proposal to an LREC, it is worth discussing it, particularly the ethics sections, with someone who can give advice on the subject. This may include someone who has had experience of submitting a proposal to that committee.

and processed so that we can match our own interpretations of the results to those of the author. This level of scrutiny and transparency of processes is rarely available in other forms of decision making.

Research also has its disadvantages and we should not feel that research is always the answer, or that poor research is better than no research; it really depends on the quality of the study in question. Overall, if we are to make use of evidence in support of the principle of evidence-based practice we must closely examine the source and quality of that evidence to ensure it stands up to scrutiny. In this respect there are more systematic methods we can use to judge the quality of research information compared to alternatives that make it the favoured option for decision making.

Having set the scene for the book, the next chapter will consider some of the essential concepts you will need in applying research to practice. This will help you with some of the language of research and key ideas that underpin research thinking. Later chapters will provide you with essential skills such as critiquing research articles (Chapter 5) and reviewing the literature (Chapter 6). You will find that each chapter ends in a similar way, applying the content of each chapter to 1. conducting research, and 2. critiquing research. Throughout, important research terms are italicised and appear in the glossary at the end of this book.

CONDUCTING RESEARCH

This book concentrates on applied research, that is, research designed to improve professional practice and clinical outcomes. Therefore, midwifery researchers, when designing new projects, should consider the relevance of their study for practice. Will midwives and women in contact with services benefit from such a study? This is neatly summed up by the challenged: *'who cares'* and *'so what'*? Therefore, the decision to carry out a study should be clearly justified and its quality equally apparent.

CRITIQUING RESEARCH

Clift-Mathews (2009) suggests that midwives need to be regular readers of research articles, and warns that without being aware of the evidence on which practice is based it is difficult to defend one's clinical decisions if scrutinised. However, the assumption is that midwives have the skills to evaluate, or critique, published research. As we shall see in Chapter 5, critiquing research is concerned with recognising how the researcher has carried out the study and having an opinion about the quality of the research. The problem is what do you need to know before you can adequately express an informed opinion? One indicator might be the extent to which the findings may help improve practice. Can the results help midwives in their clinical activities? Will it help to provide the evidence to influence clinical decisions? Can the results be transferred to other settings and geographical locations? Do they appear accurate and genuine? Here we must be mindful that it is not only the results, but the researcher's interpretation of those results, that need to be considered. Researchers who strongly believe in a particular clinical process or technique may interpret their results in a way that only sees the outcome they hoped for. In other words, the researchers must convince the reader that they were objective and had an open mind in the way in which they conducted the study. It is these kinds of questions that will be developed as you work your way through subsequent chapters.

KEY POINTS

- Midwifery services are now provided within the context of evidence-based practice. This means midwives must avoid practices based on ritual and routine, and ensure that clear and acceptable evidence supports their clinical practice.
- Evidence-based practice is compatible with the philosophy of midwifery as it seeks to provide the highest and safest levels of care. It is an ethically and professionally defendable process.
- Working within a culture of evidence-based practice demands each midwife can demonstrate a range of skills, including an understanding key research concepts and principles, as well as skills in searching the literature, critiquing articles, and synthesising research into clinical guidelines.
- This book will provide an introduction to the knowledge and skills midwives need to play an appropriate role in the generation and application of research evidence to benefit those in contact with midwifery services.

REFERENCES

Albers, L., 2001. 'Evidence' and midwifery practice. J. Midwifery and Women's Health 46 (3), 130–136.

Bluff, R., Holloway, I., 2008. The efficacy of midwifery role models. Midwifery 24 (3), 301–309.

Burns, N., Grove, S., 2009. The Practice of Nursing Research: Appraisal, Synthesis, and Generation of Evidence. sixth ed. Saunders, St. Louis.

Chalmers, I., Enkin, M., Keirse, M. (Eds.), 1989. Effective Care in Pregnancy and Childbirth. Oxford University, Oxford.

Cleary-Holdforth, J., Leufer, T., 2009. Evidence-based practice: Sowing the seeds for success. Nurse Educ. Pract. 9 (5), 285–287.

Clift-Mathews, V., 2009. Research: making the profession stronger. British Journal of Midwifery 17 (5), 276.

Cluett, E., 2005. Using the evidence to inform decisions. In: Raynor, M., Marshall, J., Sullivan, A. (Eds.), Decision Making in Midwifery Practice. Elsevier, Edinburgh.

Craig, J., 2007. How to ask the right question. In: Craig, J., Smyth, R. (Eds.), The Evidence-Based Practice Manual For Nurses. second ed.. Churchill Livingstone, Edinburgh.

Cullum, N., Ciliska, D., Haynes, R.B., Marks, S. (Eds.), 2008. Evidence-Based Nursing: An Introduction. Blackwell, Oxford.

Dale, A., 2005. Evidence-based practice: compatibility with nursing. Nurs. Stand. 19 (40), 48–53.

Department of Health, 1997. The New NHS: Modern, Dependable. Department of Health, London.

Enkin, M., Keirse, M., Chalmers, I. (Eds.), 1989. A Guide to Effective Care in Pregnancy and Childbirth. Oxford University, Oxford.

Fineout-Overholt, E., Melnyk, B., Schultz, A., 2005. Transforming Health Care from the Inside Out: Advancing Evidence-Based Practice in the 21st Century. J. Prof. Nurs. 21 (6), 335–344.

Flemming, K., 2008. Asking answerable questions. In: Cullum, N., Ciliska, D., Haynes, R.B., Marks, S. (Eds.), Evidence-Based Nursing: An Introduction. Blackwell, Oxford.

Gerrish, K., 2010. Evidence-based practice. In: Gerrish, K., Lacey, A. (Eds.),

The Research Process in Nursing, sixth ed.. Wiley-Blackwell, Chichester.

International Confederation of Midwives, 2005. Definition of the Midwife. http://www.internationalmidwives.org/Portals/5/Documentation/ICM%20Definition%20of%20the%20Midwife%202005.pdf (accessed 22.5.10).

King, F.J., 2005. A short history of evidence-based obstetric care. Best Pract. Res. Clin. Obstet. Gynaecol. 19 (1), 3–14.

Leap, N., 2009. Woman-centred or women-centred care: does it matter? British Journal of Midwifery 17 (1), 12–16.

Leufer, T., Cleary-Holdforth, J., 2009. Evidence-based practice: improving patient outcomes. Nurs. Stand. 23 (32), 35–39.

Munro, J., Spiby, H., 2010. The nature and use of evidence in midwifery care. In: Spiby, H., Munro, J. (Eds.), Evidence-Based Midwifery: Applications in Context. Wiley-Blackwell, Chichester.

Polit, D., Beck, C., 2008. Nursing Research: Generating and Assessing Evidence for Nursing Practice. eighth ed. Lippincott Williams and Wilkins, Philadelphia.

Roughley, G., 2007. What is evidence-based practice and why do we need to use it? British Journal of Midwifery 15 (4), 211.

Rycroft-Malone, J., Seers, K., Titchen, A., Harvey, G., Kitson, A., McCormack, B., 2004. What counts as evidence in evidence-based practice? J. Adv. Nurs. 47 (1), 81–90.

Sackett, D., Straus, S., Richardson, W., Rosenberg, W., Haynes, R., 2000. Evidence-Based Medicine: How To Practice and Teach EBM. second ed. Churchill Livingstone, Edinburgh.

Sackett, D.L., Richardson, W.S., Rosenberg, W., Haynes, R.B., 1997. Evidence-based medicine: How to practice and teach EBM. Churchill Livingston., New York.

Spiby, H., Munro, J., 2007. The development and peer review of evidence-based guidelines to support midwifery led care in labour. Midwifery 25 (2), 163–171.

Stewart, M., 2001. Whose evidence counts? An exploration of health professionals' perceptions of evidence-based practice, focusing on the maternity services. Midwifery 17 (4), 279–288.

Walsh, D., 2008. Research evidence and clinical expertise. Br. J. Nurs. 16 (8), 498.

Walsh, D., 2010. Reflections on running an evidence course. In: Spiby, H., Munro, J. (Eds.), Evidence-Based Midwifery: Applications in Context. Wiley-Blackwell, Chichester.

Key concepts in research

2

This chapter will examine some of the important concepts used by researchers and simplify the language by helping you to understand its meaning. The language of research can appear to be composed of 'jargon', that is, unhelpful and meaningless words. This can form a barrier to understanding research, as people resent the use of words they do not understand, particularly if they feel they are just being used for effect. However, in reality, the words are a shorthand for complex ideas, and once the most commonly used words are understood, research can take on a completely different level of understanding. The chapter will also cover some of the important issues that researchers face when demonstrating that their research is accurate and carried out to a high standard. These are called 'methodological issues'. An important starting point is to recognise that research takes many different forms; in this book we will focus specifically on research examining midwifery issues, carried out on the whole by midwives.

In Chapter 1 research was defined as the systematic collection of information using carefully designed and controlled methods that answer a specific question objectively and as accurately as possible. This definition can look similar to audit and so lead to some confusion between these two sources of information. The basic difference between the two, however, is that the key role of research is to extend knowledge and understanding of a particular topic or issue through the systematic collection of information that leads to generalisations about the topic examined. Research conclusions are usually placed within a context of existing knowledge. That is, they are usually compared to previous research that has examined the same topic in order to confirm existing knowledge or help to clarify or extend it. The purpose is always to enrich our understanding of the topic so that we can better use, or control its features.

Audit, on the other hand, is usually interested in the performance level of a part of a service, and a comparison of results against an agreed standard (or previous audit results) that may allow action to be taken. Watson and

© 2011 Elsevier Ltd. All rights reserved.

Keady (2008) suggest that we can think of audit as management activity concerned with measuring the extent to which agreed standards for clinical practice or procedures are being met or are reaching a sufficient level. Gerrish and Lacey (2010) agree, saying it is a process of measuring care against predetermined standards. This is very different from the way research is designed to increasing our overall understanding of a topic and which can be applied generally, rather than the very specific location to which audit data can apply.

One problem in trying to define research is that it is similar to words such as 'care', 'birth', or 'midwifery'; it is used as though it consisted of a single entity when, in fact, in can take many different alternative forms. This means that once we decide to study it, we have to learn something about the many forms it can take. At this stage it is useful to think of research as a process that will follow a number of principles or guidelines that will change depending on the type or category of research considered. In this book we will focus on midwifery research, that is, research that explores the problems and issues of direct concern to the midwife and that has implications for the work of the midwife more than any other discipline.

QUANTITATIVE AND QUALITATIVE RESEARCH

These two concepts are an ideal starting point for learning about research as they categorise very different approaches to thinking about the role of research and the beliefs or philosophies underpinning its production. This is important as it explains why some studies look very different from others. If we know why they differ we can make the best use of both types. Although Chapter 4 on quantitative and qualitative research explores the differences in more detail in, here we need outline ideas associated with them, and the implications these have for midwifery research and knowledge.

Historically, research has been synonymous with the word 'scientific', often associated with words like 'objective' or 'accurate', as these are two key characteristics that 'good' research is presumed to posses. Gerrish and Lacey (2010: 8) see a scientific approach to research as indicating 'a rigorous approach to a systematic form of enquiry'. The philosophy or belief on which this approach is based is that the natural or 'real' world does not depend on an individual's experience of it to exist and that it is open to study and quantification. In other words, it can be measured in some way independent of the person doing the measuring. This type of research can be characterised as *'quantitative'* research as it attempts to quantify concepts, such as blood pressure, family size and even pain, in the form of a numeric value. These numbers can be summarised and allow the use of a range of statistical techniques to give the results greater usefulness and meaning (Chapter 13). The purpose of quantitative research is seen as the search for relationships between things in the world so that we can understand the way they act and relate together. The ultimate aim of this understanding is to be able to control the elements in our world that impact on human existence. Our understanding of gravity and how we are influenced by its 'laws' is a good example of this measurement and developing of relationships leading to theories about 'how things are'. In midwifery, an example may be the search for a relationship between physical skin-to-skin contact with the baby at birth and parental feelings of emotional attachment so this pattern can be measured and demonstrated to be advantageous.

This scientific view is one *'paradigm'* or total way of looking at things (world view) in research. It is the one embraced by medical research as the 'right' and 'proper' approach for a profession that is concerned with clinical outcomes. These words have been put in inverted commas to show that there may not be total agreement on this statement, and it is open to debate whether the belief applies in all circumstances. We must remember that this is only one approach to research and, without suggesting that it is not an indispensable approach in midwifery, that there are other, just as legitimate ways of conducting a study in addition to counting or measuring something that can also extend midwifery knowledge and practice.

Qualitative research (sometimes referred to as representing a naturalistic paradigm as it avoids controlling situations) is the second in the pair of concepts that go to make up the two largest research approaches in midwifery. This has a different view of the characteristics of knowledge and the best way of conducting research to discover, extend or confirm that knowledge. It is believed that the real world can only be understood through our personal experience of it, and everything depends on how we experience and interpret that experience. This explains why some people are afraid of spiders or going to the dentist. It is a product of how people experience them, or the associations they hold for the individual. It does not mean that spiders or dentists themselves are frightening. Naturalistic or qualitative researchers believe that if we are to understand a topic we need to look at it through the eyes of those who experience it and try to understand it from their point of view. This way of thinking creates a different understanding of reality and the type of research we need to capture it accurately. This kind of research produces qualitative data in the form of verbal or written statements and dialogue, or extensive descriptions of observed human activity and behaviour. It uses methods such as interviews or observations, and information taken from documents such as diaries or health records that capture perceptions, interpretations, experiences or understanding.

One of the guiding principles of qualitative research is that it tries to capture people's thoughts and feelings in their own words. So, questionnaires with fixed-choice options would not be classed as qualitative research even though they may have tried to see things from the individual's point of view, as the list of alternative answers has been developed by the researcher. This format does not allow individuals to express ideas and answers in their own words, only in those of the researchers who have designed the alternatives and selected what they think are relevant alternatives.

An important visual distinction between quantitative and qualitative research is the presentation of data. Quantitative research will use numerical or visual forms of data presentation such as tables, bar charts and histograms (more of these in Chapter 13 on statistics). This form of data presentation is not a main feature of qualitative research, although some studies may present a table showing details of the sample, such as age, number of children, etc. It is more usual for qualitative results to avoid numbers and simply present broad theme headings and discuss the type of comments made, often with examples of direct quotations or dialogue. As will be seen in Chapter 4, these two forms of research are so different they are almost two different entities. The importance of this is that we must avoid criticising qualitative research using the criteria of a quantitative approach.

Which of these two approaches is best suited to midwifery research? The answer is, the one that is most appropriate to the question posed. If the midwifery question is one of quantity, or frequency, particularly in regard to clinical outcomes, then a quantitative approach will be appropriate; if the question is one of perceptions, understanding and interpretations, then the best approach will be qualitative.

LEVELS OF QUESTIONS IN RESEARCH

There is no shortage of questions that need to be answered through midwifery research. From the research point of view, it is the question posed by the researcher that results in the aim of the research. The aim usually begins with the word 'to' as in:

> ... this study aims to examine how a certain group of midwives (the participants) conceptualise the phenomenon of the 'good' midwife and the 'good' leader.
>
> Byrom and Downe (2010: 127)

Research questions will differ in their complexity and this will have implications for the way a study is designed. Wood and Ross-Kerr (2006) make a useful distinction between what they call the three levels of research question. These levels are influenced by how much is known about a particular subject, or how much theory exists in relation to it (Table 2.1). The advantage of this system is that it allows you to predict the way a study should be structured to answer a question at each of the levels.

- *Level-one questions* form the most basic level where very little is known about the topic. The purpose of this type of research is to describe a situation. The work of McMunn et al. (2009) is an example of this, where the purpose was to determine current use of TENS in England, to gain understanding of midwifery views on TENS use, and to establish the level

Table 2.1   Levels of research questions

Level of question	Description	Type of research
Level 1	Examines one variable (or a series of variables) but without looking for patterns between variables. Exploratory situation where little is known about the topic.	Quantitative descriptive, e.g. survey Qualitative study: all types are level 1.
Level 2	Looks for a statistical relationship between variables that are present in the form of a pattern or association.	Correlation survey where variables frequently seem to be present together, e.g. social class and likelihood to breastfeed.
Level 3	Looks for the presence of a statistical relationship between variables that indicate a cause and effect relationship, that is, an intervention always has an influence on an outcome.	Randomised control trial where the effect of an intervention is measured in terms of a clinical outcome.

of support for a randomised controlled trial of TENS versus standard care for women in labour. As can be seen, there are several aspects to this study; each part, however, is a level-one question, as the results will only answer one question at a time. As there is little known about this situation, the purpose of the study is to gain basic information on the topic. McMunn et al. (2009) answer these questions in a level-one survey and base their results on 139 (76% response rate) semi-structured questionnaires from midwives.

- *Level-two questions* are those where some basic information is known about a topic, and there is an attempt to look for a possible statistical relationship between two or more factors. An example is the study by Kerrigan and Kingdom (2010) that looked at the maternity notes of 8176 women who gave birth in one hospital. The aim of the study was to identify links between obesity and social deprivation, and compare outcomes of pregnancy in obese and non-obese women. This correlation study found that 17.7% of women were clinically obese. No correlation was found between obesity and social deprivation, but there were a number of clear correlations or links found to a number of risk factors. For example, the incidence of pre-eclampsia, gestational diabetes, induction of labour, Caesarean section and fetal macrosomia was significantly higher amongst the obese population, with all these showing a clear correlation with increase in body mass index (BMI).
- *Level-three questions* are used to test hypotheses based on already established theories about a topic. The work by McDonald et al. (2010) would be an example of this. Their randomised control trial evaluated the effectiveness of a new postnatal support package for women breastfeeding which comprised one postnatal education session and up to 6 weeks of midwifery home visits with telephone contact in comparison with a standard regimen of no extra visits (control). The study was based on the belief that early identification of breastfeeding problems and early intervention would prevent early cessation of breastfeeding. It was hypothesised that additional social support by a midwife who was an informed source of breastfeeding information would encourage women to persist with breastfeeding. A total of 849 women entered the study with 425 receiving extra support and 424 receiving standard support. It was found that there was no difference between the early cessation of breastfeeding. The conclusion was that there was already a high breastfeeding initiation rate of 87% and the factors that led to a cessation in breastfeeding were mainly social, such as a return to work.

These three levels form an important distinction, as they influence the type of approach the researcher must use to gather the data. Level-one questions require a descriptive approach, perhaps using survey methods or a qualitative approach. Level-two questions require more sophistication in the method of analysis in order to suggest that relationships between variables may exist. Finally, level-three questions require the use of an experimental approach that will test whether a hypothesis based on a theory can be supported by research evidence. Each level also requires more from those making use of the research, as the amount of research knowledge and critical analysis increases in complexity with each level.

2 VARIABLES

So far, we have already been using some of the concepts that form the basic building blocks of research. Once we are familiar with their meaning in more detail we should find our ability to analyse research has increased.

All studies are concerned with examining specified elements of interest to the researcher, such as level of pain in childbirth, intention to breastfeed, suturing skills. The term 'variable' is used to describe these items as they differ or vary in some way and can be seen to lie along a continuum. For example, length of labour, attitude towards natural childbirth methods, social class, temperature, and level of pain in labour, can vary from one person to another and can be arranged in a logical order. Burns and Grove (2009: 727) state that variables are: *'Qualities, properties, or characteristics of persons, things, or situations that change or vary and are manipulated, measured or controlled in research'*. In other words, they are the 'things' that the researcher builds the study around and so we should identify the particular variables of concern in the studies we examine.

In level-three questions involving randomised control trials, we can further subdivide variables into two types: *dependent variables* and *independent variables*. The variable that is the focus of concern, or sometimes the 'problem' the researcher is striving to improve or control, is the dependent variable, such as total length of time breastfeeding, or level of pain. The variable that is presumed to play a part in influencing the dependent variable is known as the independent variable. The independent variable can be thought of as the influencing factor or 'cause' and the dependent factor is the outcome consequence, or 'effect'.

An example will make this clear. Imagine a study whose aim is to examine whether women who have attended antenatal sessions or 'classes' are more assertive in seeking the type of birth they want than those who have not attended classes. The extent to which a woman is assertive in seeking the type of birth they want would be the dependent variable; attendance at antenatal classes would be the independent variable. Experimental research, which we shall explore later in Chapter 12, revolves around the examination of cause and effect relationships, where the researcher introduces the independent variable into the experimental group and examines its effect on outcomes.

Initially, the difference between dependent and independent variables can be difficult to grasp. An easy way of sorting them out is to think of their chronological order of measurement in an experimental study, and identify which comes first and which comes last. The variable that comes first in time is the independent variable – the influence, and the variable that comes last is the dependent variable – the outcome. In the example above, attendance at antenatal classes happens before the level of assertiveness in seeking the type of birth they want, so attendance would be the independent variable, and the level of assertiveness, the dependent variable (see Table 2.2 for more examples).

One danger in many experimental design studies is that they appear to be based on the assumption that events are influenced by only one factor. Things are rarely as simple as this, and a number of other variables may influence whether a woman is assertive at the birth. Other factors in the example of

Table 2.2 *Examples of dependent and independent variables identified from the aim of a study*

Aim	Dependent variable	Independent variable
To investigate an education discharge plan that included information about postnatal depression to reduce the severity of depression after childbirth (Ho et al. 2009)	Level of postpartum depression	Discharge education on postnatal depression provided by postpartum ward nurses
To evaluate the effects of an extended midwifery support (EMS) programme on the proportion of women who breastfeed fully to 6 months. (McDonald et al. 2010)	Proportion of women breastfeeding fully to 6 months	An extended midwifery support (EMS) programme
To evaluate the effect of active management of the third stage of labour on the amount of blood loss in the third and fourth stages of labour, and the duration of the third stage of labour (Kashanian et al. 2010)	1) the amount of blood loss in the third and fourth stages of labour, 2) the duration of the third stage of labour	The type of management of the third stage of labour (active versus 'expectant' or 'hands-off' approach)

assertiveness above include influences such as personality, the quality of the relationship with their birth partner, level of education and social class. These would also be independent variables that the researcher may need to consider in the interpretation of the results. In experimental studies, then, we should identify the dependent variable and the independent variable, and ask ourselves, 'is there anything else that could have influenced the outcome that has not been taken into account'? If we do this, then we are becoming more critical users of research.

CONCEPT DEFINITIONS AND OPERATIONAL DEFINITIONS

These two concepts explain firstly what the researcher means by the words used to describe the study variables, and secondly, how they were measured in the study. The *concept definition* is a clear statement of the sense in which the researcher is using the words describing the concept. It is similar in some ways to a dictionary definition of the word. In our example of attendance at antenatal classes and feelings of involvement, although we may feel we do not need to define the words 'antenatal classes', there are a variety of terms used to describe them in the UK, and they may well not mean the same to readers from other countries. We would also be concerned about the concept definition of what qualifies as 'attendance at classes'. If someone attended just one or two sessions are they referred to as having attended in the same way as those who have attended more times? The other term we would want clearly defined would be 'level of assertiveness'. What exactly does this mean? To provide an answer, criteria may be provided that specifies what counts as an instance of assertiveness.

The meaning of the term *operational definition* is important from the data-gathering point of view, as it indicates how a particular concept is to be measured or *'operationalised'*. Houser (2008: 245) define the operational definition as *'an explanation of the procedures that must be performed to accurately represent the concepts'*. In other words, how we go about converting the variable into some numeric value, whether that is by means of a scale or a scoring system. So, for instance, the condition of the baby following birth may be operationalised using the Apgar score, and this converts the condition of the baby at birth and will permit the condition of different babies to be compared accurately. Concepts such as pain and anxiety, are now operationalised using a scale that is regarded as a reasonably objective measure. For example, participants may be asked to mark on a 100-mm line how sever their symptoms have been for health problems they may have experienced. This calibrated line is known as a visual analogue scale (VAS) and is used to operationalise concepts that do not usually have a numeric value attached to them. The line is divided into 25-mm sections so that the location of a cross, indicated by a respondent along the line, can be given a numeric value, and comparisons made between respondents.

THEORETICAL AND CONCEPTUAL FRAMEWORKS

One of the aims of research is to add to the body of knowledge on a particular subject, and to increase understanding by developing a more accurate theory about why things happen the way they do. A particular study cannot look at everything and will confine itself to a number of key factors or variables. The researcher's understanding of those variables can be expressed in terms of the theoretical framework that is adopted for the study. This provides a clear context for the study. Burns and Grove (2009: 725) define a theory as *'an integrated set of defined concepts and existence statements, and relational statements that present a view of a phenomenon and can be used to describe, explain, predict or control that phenomenon'*. This gives the theoretical framework an important place in research as it guides the thinking of the researcher and provides the study with a specific context. So, for instance, the principle to provide a mother, and often the father, with skin-to-skin contact with the newborn baby is based on the theory of parental attachment. This would be used in a study to construct a hypothesis, for instance, that mothers and fathers who have skin-to-skin contact with their babies will show higher levels of bonding with their baby and spend more time interacting with the baby following the birth than those who do not have skin-to-skin contact. The theory will also be used to identify what information should be collected as part of the data collected to test the theory.

The relationship between concepts is sometimes presented diagrammatically to illustrate how the author visualises the links between the dependent and independent variable(s). These diagrams are sometimes referred to as conceptual frameworks or conceptual maps, where key concepts are joined by lines and arrows to show the direction and nature of the relationships believed to exist. So a study may concentrate on the concept of breastfeeding, and be concerned with some of the independent variables, which may influence the adoption of breastfeeding. A suitable conceptual framework that would illustrate the researcher's thinking may look something like Figure 2.1.

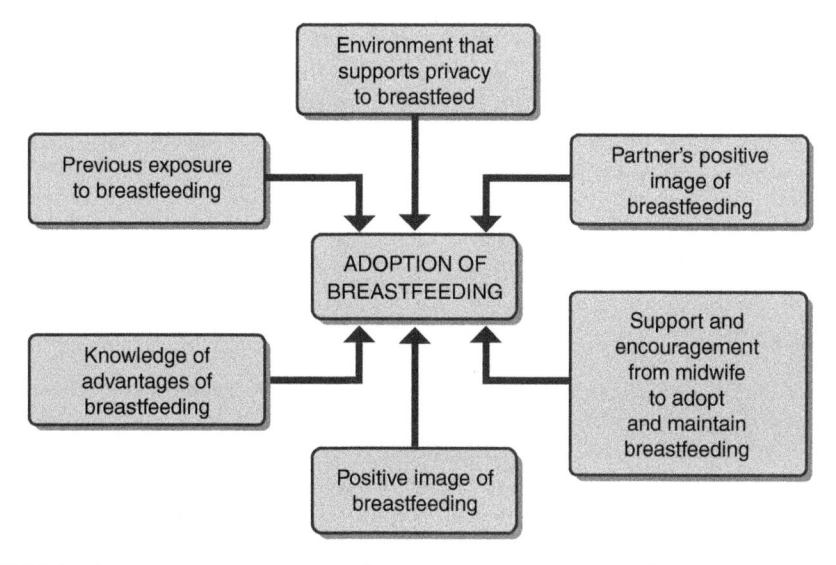

FIG 2.1 Conceptual framework for a study exploring the decision to breastfeed.

As can be seen, conceptual frameworks provide a mental image of what the researcher sees as the influencing factors or variables that will be explored in a study. This provides the researcher with a clear picture of the topic area and should influence the design of the study, the key concepts, the elements included in the tool of data collection and the analysis and interpretation of data. In other words, they are a very powerful part of a research process. It is for this reason that a thorough review of the literature is essential to provide the theoretical and conceptual context for the study. This will then provide a clear indication of the key concepts that require concept and operational definitions.

One final word is to emphasise that the use of theories and conceptual frameworks do vary between quantitative research, which will usually start with a theory and conceptual framework, and qualitative research, which is more likely to develop one during or following data analysis. Remember, not all studies will explicitly include a theoretical or conceptual framework.

RELIABILITY, VALIDITY, BIAS AND RIGOUR

These four concepts are amongst the most valuable to use when critiquing research as they form part of the language that allows studies to be evaluated in terms of their design and way they are carried out. The words themselves may be familiar but their exact meaning may be unclear. The first two, reliability and validity, are used mainly when discussing quantitative research approaches and are concerned with the nature of measurement.

RELIABILITY

This relates to the method of collecting data and refers to the accuracy and consistency of the measurements produced by the tool of data collection.

For example, if we wanted to carpet a room, the use of a metre length of elastic to measure the area would make us distrust the reliability of the method of collecting the measurements. Reliability then, relates to the consistency and accuracy of the measurement tool. If a study involved weighing babies as part of data collection, we would want to ensure any weighing scales used were tested for accuracy. Where a number of different scales were used we would want to ensure that each one gave an accurate reading, otherwise the reliability of the results would be open to question.

VALIDITY

This relates to what is being measured and is an attempt to ensure that the research tool is really measuring what the researcher believes it is measuring. So, for instance, we could think we were looking at the satisfaction of women with the clinical skills of their midwife, when we were really measuring the influence of the midwife's personality that may influence how women felt about the care they received. Although reliability is usually amenable to checking, and may become apparent in a pilot study, validity is far more difficult to confirm.

BIAS

The degree of accuracy in the results of a study will be influenced by the amount of *bias* contained in the research. Bias has been defined by Polit and Beck (2008) as *'an influence that produces a distortion or error in the study results'* (p. 197). This can take a number of different forms, as we shall see in later sections. Here, we will concentrate on bias within the sample that may make them untypical or unrepresentative of the group they represent (see Chapter 14). This can happen through the method of sample selection.

In describing the sample, the researcher frequently mentions the *inclusion and exclusion criteria* used to select those in the study. These terms relate to the characteristics of those felt to be typical of the study group – the inclusion criteria, and those characteristics that were felt may either put them at clinical risk, or that would introduce bias into the group – the exclusion criteria. It is important to examine these closely and assess whether you feel the researcher has attempted to control for bias in the way the sample were selected. Look, too, for any changes in the size of the groups as a result of people not completing a study once they had started (this is called the mortality rate). This may make comparisons between groups difficult, as they may no longer be similar in composition once a number of people have dropped out of the study. The results will be distorted by the fact that although the two groups may have been comparable at the start, they are not at the end when a number from one of the groups did not complete the study.

RIGOUR

This is the final of the four major concept used to assess studies and relates to the overall planning and implementation of the research design. It examines whether the researcher has carried out the study in a logical, systematic way and paid attention to factors that may influence the accuracy of the results. Burns and Grove (2009: 34) suggest that rigour is the *'striving for excellence in research and involves discipline, scrupulous adherence to detail, and strict accuracy'*. They argue that a rigorously conducted study has precise measurement tools, a representative sample and a tightly controlled study design. They also make the point that rigour applies just as much to qualitative research as to quantitative, where poorly developed methods, inadequate time spent gathering and analysing the data can all negatively affect the quality of the research, as we shall see in Chapter 4.

Having examined these key concepts, we can see that midwifery has a body of knowledge that draws on both quantitative and qualitative research approaches. The issues and problems faced in research relate both to the worlds of quantification found in the scientific approach, and the naturalistic world as experienced by those who come into contact with midwifery services, including midwives themselves. This book is concerned with this wide spectrum of research approaches and illustrates the knowledge of research required to make the best use of studies that can play a major role in providing evidence-based practice.

CONDUCTING RESEARCH

The key research concepts included in this chapter are essential to the researcher at the planning stage of a project. Understanding these concepts and the relationships between them will enable researchers to plan their study in such a way that it will stand up to scrutiny. Together, they provide a basic vocabulary not only to plan a study but also provide the researcher with possible ways of reducing the inevitable problems that are part of any study.

CRITIQUING RESEARCH

Research articles can appear to be written in a foreign language unless the reader has a basic understanding of the concepts introduced in this chapter. Once these have been absorbed, the reader will not only understand far more, but will become more appreciative of good research, and sensitive to weak research.

Knowing the distinction between quantitative and qualitative research will help anticipate the appropriate research approach, and the type of data collected. As will be seen in Chapter 5, there are two different approaches to critiquing an article depending on whether it is quantitative or qualitative in design.

An ability to identify the level of the research question will allow the reader to make certain assumptions about the research and the form it takes. Knowledge of the levels also provides a way of critically examining the study to ensure that the researcher has considered the implications of the different levels, and has not introduced something that is inappropriate to that level.

In reading a research report, a reader should quickly establish the variables under scrutiny. The clarity of the concept and operational definitions will ensure the reader knows exactly what the researcher is examining and how it is measured. Where the question is level three, the reader should identify the dependent and independent variables in order to follow the outcome measure that forms the dependent variable, and what the researcher introduces in the form of the independent variable.

The underlying theoretical or conceptual framework will also allow the reader to understand why the particular elements have been linked and the underlying assumptions made by the researcher. In identifying the theoretical or conceptual framework, the reader should ensure that the items in the tool of data collection and the discussion of the findings reflect the theoretical or conceptual framework.

Critiquing is about assessing how well the researcher has accomplished the design and presentation of their research. It is an assessment of both the strengths and weakness of a written or verbal research presentation. In order to provide a fair assessment, the reader must always keep the concepts of reliability, validity, bias and rigour in mind. These concepts provide an informed approach to assessing, firstly, the quality of the research, and secondly, the degree of excellence achieved by the researcher.

KEY POINTS

- Research is a lot easier to appreciate through an understanding of some of the concepts covered in this chapter.
- Quantitative and qualitative approaches to research relate to the different research designs, and are based on philosophical beliefs about the nature of empirical evidence, that is, evidence collected in the real world through the senses. Quantitative research is based on the belief that the truth of a situation exists in an objective state outside the personal views or perceptions of the individual. It emphasises accuracy, and produces numerical data. Qualitative researchers believe that the truth of a situation is produced by our subjective experience, and that we need to look at things from an individual's point of view. Midwifery is concerned with issues that draw on both beliefs.
- Research questions can relate to three levels of exploration. Level-one questions relate to describing one variable, usually about which little is known, or that has rarely been the subject of research. Level-two questions look for relationships between variables but where little theory exists. Level-three questions relate to questions where theory exists and the aim is to test hypotheses based on the theory.
- Variables are the elements in which the researcher is interested. In level-three questions, there will be a dependent variable that is the outcome or effect, and one or more independent variables that are presumed to influence or cause the dependent variable.
- Concept definitions relate to how the researcher defines the topic in which they are interested. This can be thought of as a dictionary definition or alternative word for the topic of interest.
- Operational definitions refer to the way in which a concept is measured. It reduces the vagueness of such words as comfort, pain, and benefit by producing a clear specification of how the researcher will make them visible in a specific study.

- Theoretical and conceptual frameworks provide the context and meaning for the ideas and concepts contained in a study.
- Reliability, validity, bias and rigour relate first to the extent to which the tool of data collection is accurate and consistent between different measurements, or different researchers. Validity relates to whether the method does measure what the researcher intends it to measure. Bias is the extent to which the findings are distorted either by the choice of subjects or the method of measurement. Rigour is the extent to which the researcher has attempted to conduct the study to ensure accuracy and high-quality research.

REFERENCES

Burns, N., Grove, S., 2009. The Practice of Nursing Research: Appraisal, Synthesis, and Generation of Evidence, sixth ed. Saunders, St Louis.

Byrom, S., Downe, S., 2010. 'She sort of shines': midwives' accounts of 'good' midwifery and 'good' leadership. Midwifery 26 (1), 126–137.

Gerrish, K., Lacey, A., 2010. Research and development in nursing. In: Gerrish, K., Lacey, A. (Eds.), The Research Process in Nursing sixth ed., Wiley-Blackwell, Chichester.

Ho, S., Hey, S., Jevitt, C., Huang, L., Fu, Y., Wang, L., 2009. Effectiveness of a discharge education program in reducing the severity of postpartum depression: A randomized controlled evaluation study. Patient Educ. Couns. 77 (1), 68–71.

Houser, J., 2008. Nursing Research: Reading, Using, and Creating Evidence. Jones and Bartlett, Boston.

Kashanian, M., Fekrat, M., Masoomi, Z., Ansari, N., 2010. Comparison of active and expectant management on the duration of the third stage of labour and the amount of blood loss during the third and fourth stages of labour: a randomised controlled trial. Midwifery 26 (2), 241–245.

Kerrigan, A., Kingdom, C., 2010. Maternal obesity and pregnancy: a retrospective study. Midwifery 26 (1), 138–146.

McDonald, S., Henderson, J., Faulkner, S., Evans, S., Hagan, R., 2010. Effect of an extended midwifery postnatal support programme on the duration of breastfeeding: A randomised controlled trial. Midwifery 26 (1), 88–100.

McMunn, V., Bedwell, C., Neilson, J., Jones, A., Dowswell, T., Lavender, T., 2009. A national survey of the use of TENS in labour. British Journal of Midwifery 17 (8), 492–495.

Polit, D., Beck, C., 2008. Nursing Research: Generating and Assessing Evidence for Nursing Practice, eighth ed. Lippincott Williams and Wilkins, Philadelphia.

Watson, R., Keady, J., 2008. The Nature and language of nursing research. In: Watson, R., McKenna, H., Cowman, S., Keady, J. (Eds.), Nursing Research: Designs and Methods. Churchill Livingstone, Edinburgh.

Wood, M., Ross-Kerr, J., 2006. Basic Steps in Planning Nursing Research: From question to Proposal, sixth ed. Jones and Bartlett, Boston.

The basic framework of research

An understanding of the basic framework of research projects is imperative, whether you are carrying out research or reading research articles. This chapter will outline the stages involved in designing and carrying out research. The framework used here applies mainly to quantitative research projects. Although qualitative research follows similar steps, the order of the stages may be different. The next chapter will provide more detail on the distinction between these two approaches.

How does a researcher carry out a research study? The answer to this question will provide you with a roadmap to understand the way the many stages in research all fit together. Before looking at the detail, we can begin our journey through the research process by looking at the broad phases of any research project, as suggested by Polit and Beck (2008: 64):

- *The Conceptual Phase* This is the main thinking phase where the researcher develops the idea for the research, and gradually develops a researchable question.
- *The Design and Planning Phase* In this phase, decisions on the broad research approach and the tool of data collection are decided.
- *The Empirical Phase* The activity part, involving the collection of information, also includes the pilot study, which tests the method.
- *The Analytic Phase* Here, the data are analysed and a report written.
- *The Dissemination Phase* Finally, the research report is communicated in the form of a report, article, conference poster or presentation so that practice can benefit from this new knowledge.

These phases can be simplified even further to a sandwich of:

THINKING – DOING – THINKING

We can see from this that research is based on thinking things through and interpreting the consequences of the information that has been collected. This has very close parallels with clinical work where we think about how to provide for the needs of the individual, action the plan and then assess how successful it has been. Research and clinical thinking, then, are not that far apart.

© 2011 Elsevier Ltd. All rights reserved.

> **BOX 3.1 Stages in the research process**
>
> 1. Develop the research question.
> 2. Critically evaluate the relevant literature.
> 3. Plan the method of investigation to include:
>   a. The broad approach i.e. quantitative or qualitative,
>   b. The sample, sample size, and sampling strategy,
>   c. The information to be gathered,
>   d. The tool of data collection,
>   e. The method of data analysis and presentation,
>   f. The ethical issues to be addressed,
>   g. Apply for funding and ethical approval.
> 4. Carry out a pilot study (if quantitative).
> 5. Collect the data.
> 6. Analyse the results.
> 7. Develop conclusions and recommendations.
> 8. Communicate the study.

We can now break down the broad phases outlined above and concentrate on each of the stages within them. The overall structure of the research process is summarised in Box 3.1.

STAGE ONE: THE RESEARCH QUESTION

Research begins when the researcher decides to examine a particular topic or answer an important question. Where do ideas for research come from? Perhaps one of the most common sources is a known problem in the practice area. The researcher's first task is to take the problem and write the research question, or *'terms of reference'*. This is a clear statement of the aim of the project. Atkinson (2008) emphasises that the role of the research question is absolutely central to the development of successful research, and so a great deal of effort is placed on getting it right. At the preliminary stage, the researcher may think in terms of a question that they want to answer that begins with 'why' 'what' 'when' or 'how'? Wood and Ross-Kerr (2006) call these words the stem of the question and what comes after them, the topic. An example would be *'what* are the factors that influence women to give up breastfeeding?' or *'who* is likely to decide on a home birth?' Giving up breastfeeding, and deciding on a home birth would be the topics and *'what'* and *'who'* would be the stem.

These questions are then converted into the research aim by removing the stem and replacing it with *'to identify'*, *'to compare'*, *'to determine'* or a similar phrase. So, for instance, we could say the aim of our study was 'to identify the factors that influence women to give up breastfeeding', or 'to determine the characteristics of women who are likely to decide on a home birth'. Table 3.1 illustrates questions that have been developed into research aims.

In experimental and some correlation studies, the researcher will usually state a *hypothesis*, or even more than one. A hypothesis has been defined by

Table 3.1 *Research questions and aims*

Author	Question	Research aim
Byrom and Downe (2010)	What are the characteristics regarded as making a 'good' midwife and good leader?	To examine how a certain group of midwives (the participants) conceptualise the phenomenon of the 'good' midwife and the 'good' leader.
Jackson and Fraser (2009)	What knowledge and attitudes do midwives have in relation to caring for women who have been sexually abused?	To investigate midwives' knowledge and attitudes in relation to caring for women who have been sexually abused.
Hindley et al. (2008)	How much choice are women given about intrapartum monitoring of the fetal heart?	To investigate the degree of choice pregnant women at low obstetric risk had in making informed decisions on the use of intrapartum fetal monitoring techniques.

Schmidt and Brown (2009: 64) as a formal statement regarding the expected or predicted relationship between two or more variables in a specific population. In more simple terms, it is the 'hunch' that the researcher has about the outcome of the study. In experimental studies, the aim is to predict the nature of the relationship between the independent and dependent variables.

Although a hypothesis is not required in descriptive research, as the purpose is not to test the relationship between variables, it is sometimes helpful for the researcher to consider what assumptions they have about influencing factors. These can be used in deciding what information to gather. So in describing what attracts some women to a home birth and not others, the researcher might hypothesise that factors such as social class, age and parity may be influential. These would then be included as questions in the tool of data collection.

An important consideration at this stage is whether the question is researchable. This relates firstly to the practical aspect of the study in terms of whether it is the kind of question that could be tackled by research reasonably easily – what Punch (2006) refers to as whether it is feasible and 'doable'? Secondly, it is important to realise that not all questions are amenable to investigation. Philosophical questions, or ethical issues, cannot be answered through research. Such questions as 'should midwives wear a uniform' or 'should midwives reserve the right to strike' belong in this category and are really the subjects of debate, not research.

The first stage of research is complex. The type and nature of the question are important, not only from the professional point of view of do we need to know the answer, but also in relation to the research method. Many of the other stages in the research process will be influenced by the way the aim is written. So, for instance, the broad approach, the method of data collection, the sample and method of data analysis can all be implicitly influenced by the aim of the study.

STAGE TWO: REVIEWING THE LITERATURE

Studies are not undertaken in isolation from previous research; therefore the second stage of the research process consists of a critical review of current literature on the topic. The purpose of this is to gain more information about the topic being examined. The literature also helps to clarify the research question and possible ways of answering it (see Chapter 7). It also confirms that there is a need for such a study. As Lacey (2010) points out, there is no point in carrying out research if the question has already been competently answered. Although this stage is an essential element in quantitative research, in qualitative research the literature is not always consulted at this point; instead it is used at the analysis stage to help make sense of the data. Qualitative researchers sometimes avoid examining the literature too early in case their own views are influenced by what they read, and so restrict the topics and issues included in data collection and analysis.

In quantitative research, reviewing the literature is an important part of clarifying one's ideas, and a necessary early stage in the research process, particularly in justifying the need for such a study. Midwifery is extremely fortunate in having such resources as the MIDIRS information system and the Cochrane Collaboration database available to access information on published midwifery research. Accessing databases through local midwifery and nursing libraries and on-line resources are also part of the process of gathering information on previous studies (Chapter 6).

The review is important not only to provide information on the topic, but also to provide guidance on the approach and methods used by those who have studied a particular topic previously. The 'methods' section of research articles provides useful guidance on the way data can be gathered in a study and any possible pitfalls that might be attached to some methods. Most authors provide some details of problems encountered and comment on what they would have done differently with hindsight. All these are valuable to the researcher planning a study. Once this stage is reached, it is worth the researcher stopping and asking the following three questions:

- Does it need to be done, or should practice be based on the research evidence already available?
- What use will be made of the results? Are the results likely to influence practice?
- Can I do it? Do I have the resources, skills and time for this to be carried out rigorously?

Unless the answers to these questions are in the positive, there may be little point in moving on to the next stage of planning the study.

STAGE THREE: PLANNING THE STUDY

Once the first two stages are complete, the researcher is ready to plan the study from beginning to end. The quality of the research will be influenced by the amount of preparation and planning that have been invested in the process. Rigour is an important aspect in research and is dependent on this thinking phase. As was seen in Chapter 2, rigour involves the researcher attempting to produce the highest-quality study. This is achieved by considering possible problems that may be encountered and planning to reduce them as far as possible. Box 3.1 lists the considerations that should be included in this planning stage.

THE RESEARCH DESIGN

This is the outline of the process the researcher will follow and is influenced by the purpose of the research. If the researcher aims to establish cause-and-effect relationships, as in a level-three question (see Chapter 2), then the research approach would be experimental. If the purpose is to describe a situation, as in a level-one question, then a descriptive approach would be appropriate, perhaps using a survey method. A survey may also be used where the researcher wishes to identify if certain variables are related, as in a level-two question that looks at correlation.

There are other approaches, such as action research, where the action researcher is seen as the facilitator and evaluator of change (Meyer 2010). This has not become a widely used approach in midwifery, and there are few clear examples of its use. Its emphasis on change makes it appealing to those who want to develop clinical practice, and the involvement of those working in the areas involved in change in its design and implementation is a strong feature. This level of local involvement avoids the introduction of change for its own sake, and ensures that any developments demonstrate benefits over the current situation. Meyer (2010) does highlight that it differs from other research approaches in that there is a blurring of the boundaries between education, practice and research. To be truly a research approach, it should contribute to increasing our understanding or have the potential to be 'theory generating', which Waterman and Hope (2008) suggest is what distinguishes it from other forms of change strategies, audit and evidence-based practice.

An example of its use is the study by McKeller et al. (2008) which set out to improve postnatal education for parents, especially fathers, in Adelaide, Australia. As is typical of the action research structure, there were a number of phases to the study including questionnaires to parents, a working group of staff, including a fatherhood support worker, and the use of focus groups with fathers. The result was a more 'father-friendly' approach to postnatal education and the production of 'father postcards' to provide father-specific information.

Historic research is another method that has had only limited application within midwifery, despite the potential for providing a sense of development within the profession. It relies on the use of historical records and accounts, such as diaries, to chart the course of a particular issue or problem. The work of Allotey (2009) provides some guidelines for conducting this type of research and the dangers of misinterpreting the past.

Finally, audit should be mentioned despite not being a research approach, as the use of audit in midwifery has become so common as part of the process of evidence-based practice that it merits inclusion here. Audit often looks like research, and certainly requires the same systematic approach and rigour found in research. However, its purpose is not to add to midwifery knowledge, nor can the results of one audit be applied elsewhere; yet it does answer important questions that are very similar to level-one research questions in terms of the level of performance within a maternity service against a standard.

THE SAMPLE

The sample is the term used to describe the people, items, or events included in a study (see Chapter 14). In the planning stage the researcher must consider the characteristics that make individuals eligible for selection, and those that would make them unsuitable or even put them at risk or at a disadvantage. These considerations form the *inclusion and exclusion criteria* of a study. The researcher should also attempt to estimate the intended size of the sample when drawing up the research proposal for an ethics committee or funding body, as the sample size will both affect the credibility of the study and have consequences for funding. Comparisons with previous research may provide some clue as to optimum size, as well as helping with the sampling method.

DECIDING ON THE DATA TO BE COLLECTED

In any study it is important to avoid collecting information simply for the sake of it, in the belief that everything is relevant and should be included. This will result in information overload and make it difficult to do anything with the findings, as well as increasing costs related to processing the information. The researcher should consider each item of information to be included and ask two questions:

- Is this relevant to my research aim?
- What use am I going to make of this information?

Unless both of these can be clearly answered, the information should not be included.

THE METHOD OF DATA COLLECTION

There are a number of alternative tools of data collection that can be used to gather information. Those most frequently used include:

- questionnaires,
- interviews,
- observation,
- documentary methods,
- clinical measurements (scales, physiological measures related to clinical outcomes).

Each one will have its advantages and disadvantages, so how does a researcher know which one to choose? One of the main considerations in selecting the data collection tool is the research aim. If the research question is related to staff or women's experiences, views and opinions, and they are in the best position to provide an answer, then questionnaires or interviews will be appropriate. Where the researcher is interested in behaviour or techniques, such as methods of conducting antenatal classes, then observation will be a more reliable method. This is true of any question where we are concerned with what people do, rather than with what people say they do. Remember, too, that much of our behaviour and actions are carried out at a subconscious level, so we may find it difficult to accurately describe what we do. For everyday quantitative data, midwifery notes or the medical record may be the best source of information. Finally, where we are carrying out a level-three study where we want to establish the possible existence of cause-and-effect relationships, we would use clinical measurements, including physiological measurements or scales that will accurately quantify the outcome we are examining.

It is possible to use more than one method of collecting data in a single study to cross-check the accuracy of the information gathered and this is one form of *triangulation*. The term is used to describe the combination of alternative elements in research to examine the same variable. Here we are using it to describe combining information from different tools of data collection examining the same variable, but Burns and Grove (2009: 231) point out triangulation can describe the combination of two or more theories, methods, sources of data, researchers, or analysis methods in a single study. Each of these is used for the same purpose, which is to overcome the limitations of a single method of collecting data and so increase the validity of the results or its interpretation. As part of triangulation related to data collection, researchers might interview midwives on how they discuss smoking in pregnancy with mothers, and then observe interactions to provide a more complete and accurate picture of what goes on.

THE METHOD OF ANALYSIS AND PRESENTATION

Whichever tool is selected to gather the data, the method of analysis should be considered at the design stage, not after the data are collected. If the analysis will involve the use of statistical methods, then the researcher must decide which ones would be most appropriate and the form in which the data would need to be collected (see Chapter 13). Frequently, the researcher would consult a statistician or someone who can provide appropriate advice. At this stage it is also important to think how the numeric results will be presented, for example, in tables, graphs, or other form of display. This will also include thinking how different variables in the study may be combined in the form of cross-tabulation where one variable is subdivided by another variable. An example would be where the method of infant feeding is to be presented by parity. The method of analysis will also influence the form in which the information is collected. If the researcher wants to provide an analysis of the average length of time babies were breastfed, it would be necessary to ask women for the time in weeks and not ask them to tick a box that related to a spread of weeks, for example 3–6 or 7–10 weeks, as averages are calculated using specific numbers and not a broad range.

ETHICAL ISSUES

Just as the midwife is bound by a professional code of conduct, so the researcher is bound by an ethical code in conducting research. Ethics in research relate to a number of issues concerned with the correct behaviour and processes followed by the researcher and include the following:

- informed consent,
- confidentiality,
- the avoidance of harm or exposure to risk,

- the avoidance of raising expectations that it may not be possible to meet,
- the approval of a research ethics committee (REC) as part of research governance.

All of these issues are covered in more detail in Chapter 8. At the planning stage, the researcher must consider the implications of the study for each of these issues and plan for how they will be addressed during the study. These details are then highlighted when applying for ethical approval.

Once the planning stage is complete the researcher may be required to produce a research proposal. This is a written outline of the study and includes the justification for the study, the aim and many of the details developed in the planning phase. It will also contain a costing for the whole study and estimation of the time scale and numbers of staff to complete the study. The research proposal may be used to gain permission to undertake the study and apply for funding or submitted to the ethics committee, if appropriate, to gain ethical approval or to a scientific scrutiny panel to consider the methods being proposed. The importance of gaining this kind of permission and support means that the researcher must demonstrate the ability to complete the work involved. The proposal also allows the researcher to assess the how well all the aspects of the study will fit together. This may reveal some aspects of the study that had not been previously considered.

STAGE FOUR: PILOT

Before the study is carried out, the researcher must ensure that there are few unanticipated problems in gaining access to the data, and that the method used to collect the data will work. This is the role of the pilot study. Houser (2008: 356) describes a pilot as an intentionally smaller version of a study with a limited sample size or group of measures where the primary purpose is to test the methods and procedures of a study before the full implementation of a study. Although its purpose usually relates to assessing the accuracy of the data collection tool, it should be used to consider a range of factors. These include the whole feasibility of the study in terms of the resources, time, availability of subjects, their willingness to participate and the support required from others to facilitate data collection. All these need to be assessed before a total and perhaps expensive commitment to the study is made.

The results gathered in the pilot should also be analysed to test the way they will be processed in the main study. The major outcome of the pilot will be the assessment of the reliability of the data collection tool and the opportunity to practise using it. Refinements can then be made that will allow the main study to progress as efficiently as possible. In this respect, the pilot study is very much like a dress rehearsal that allows all the elements in the study to be tested and adjustments made before the opening night.

STAGE FIVE: DATA COLLECTION

Once the pilot had been completed, the researcher is ready to start data collection. As can be seen, this comes quite some way into the total process. Despite attempts to reduce problems, unexpected things do go wrong. For example, postal strikes happen once questionnaires have been sent out and delay their return, sickness and absence reduce the number of people available for interview, and newspapers and television influence respondents by suddenly promoting the very topic being examined in the study. All this is inevitable and a normal part of the research process.

STAGE SIX: DATA ANALYSIS

This is the stage in the research process which, according to Lacey (2010), is the most demanding from an intellectual point of view as it relates to firstly grouping the data so that they can be examined and secondly to interpreting the data that is sound and logical. Data analysis takes place when the data have been collected. Descriptive statistics may be used to present a picture of the results using techniques such as averages which can take the form of the 'mean', 'mode' or 'median' (Polit and Beck 2008: 563). Terms such as these will be explained in Chapter 13. Statistical tests or correlation may be used to establish if there are any statistical associations present. In qualitative research the vast amount of information collected is analysed to establish themes and categories. These are then compared with the literature to achieve greater validity of the findings, and to help in theory construction. The process is very complex but, as with statistical analysis, follows a systematic orderly and systematic approach (Holloway and Wheeler 2010). The exact form of analysis will vary with the type of qualitative design used. In many instances, special computer programs are available to examine some aspects of the data, although a great deal of the analysis and interpretation is carried out by the researcher. Once the data have been 'ordered' in some way, the researcher has then to interpret them so that an answer to the research question can be established.

STAGE SEVEN: CONCLUSIONS AND RECOMMENDATIONS

The data analysis should lead to conclusions. These should be based on and supported by the results. The conclusion should also provide an answer to the aim of the study, and, where appropriate, say whether the study hypothesis has been accepted or rejected. (We do not say proved or disproved because there is always a margin of error.) The implications of the findings are then discussed and will result in recommendations both for further research and for changes in practice where appropriate.

STAGE EIGHT: COMMUNICATION OF FINDINGS

Research will only be useful if it is communicated. The last stage in the research process consists of the production of a report, article or verbal presentation where the author will provide the following details:

- what they set out to do (aim),
- why they did it (rationale),
- how they did it (methodology),
- what they found (results),
- what it all means (discussion and recommendations).

We can now use this knowledge of the research process in Chapter 5, which covers critiquing research. Further chapters will look at some of the topics and issues covered in this chapter in more detail.

CONDUCTING RESEARCH

This chapter has presented the basic framework the researcher follows in carrying out research. This framework is very methodical and has an internal consistency where every stage has implications for further stages. Although it is presented here as a series of steps, it should be acknowledged that some of these are carried out in parallel, or the researcher may go back to certain stages and carry out further work on them. It is not necessarily as neat as it appears.

The essence of good research is planning, and the researcher will increase the chances of a successful project the more time that is spent on this stage. The importance of the review of the literature is not only to provide a context for the study, but also to guide the way the study will be conducted. This includes influencing the questions included in the data collection tool. Above all, the researcher should not be tempted to economise by neglecting a pilot study, as so many unanticipated problems can be revealed at this stage.

The practical feasibility of the study should be carefully considered, and two important elements at the planning stage are, firstly, to think about permission to conduct the study, and secondly, to design the method of data analysis, whether this involves statistics or qualitative data analysis. Where the study will clearly need ethical approval, it is worth contacting the appropriate Research Ethics Committee (REC) as soon as possible, as failure to do so can seriously delay a study. There can also be other stages involved before the ethics committee, such as a scientific scrutiny panel that will first assess whether the proposed method is sound and completing an online submission to the National Research Ethics Service (NRES). A research proposal, which is the outline of the intended research, will have to be submitted to these various groups, so get advice from someone who has experience in this. Similarly, at this stage advice should be sought from someone who has an understanding of statistics or the analysis of qualitative data. The method of data analysis will have a profound effect on the type and format of the information included in the data collection tool. A mistake at this point could mean that a large part of the information collected is unusable because it has not been collected in the right format.

Although researchers can spend a great deal of time on planning, and even on piloting the study, inevitably things do not always run smoothly, and the unexpected might well happen to you. Research is a skill acquired through experience over time. However, do not give up when things go wrong – adjust your plan and move on.

CRITIQUING RESEARCH

The research process framework provided in this chapter gives a useful structure to use in evaluating or critiquing published research. As you read through a study there should be clear evidence that the stages in the research process have been followed, and the issues outlined in this section addressed. If they have not, then you are justified to question the rigour of the study. Remember, however, that qualitative research has a different structure, and will look different in comparison to quantitative research reports. More details on this will appear in the next chapter.

The important question when critiquing a study is *'has the researcher followed a sensible plan of action given the nature of the research question'*? The next question should be, *'does each decision fit with the previous decision made in the process'*? Once you are familiar with the stages of research you will see the structure clearly evident in all the reports you read.

KEY POINTS

- Research projects are structured according to a number of stages that provide the researcher with a path to follow. The aim of this framework is to increase objectivity, reliability, validity and the rigour of the research.
- The exact sequence of steps will vary depending on the broad research design. Qualitative research is different in structure and process from quantitative research.
- Knowing these steps enables the reader of a research project to assess whether the correct stages have been followed.

REFERENCES

Allotey, J., 2009. Writing midwives' history: problems and pitfalls. Midwifery doi: 10.1016/j.midw.2009.03.003.

Atkinson, I., 2008. Asking research questions. In: Watson, R., McKenna, H., Cowman, S., Keady, J. (Eds.), Nursing Research: Designs and Methods. Churchill Livingstone, Edinburgh.

Burns, N., Grove, S., 2009. The Practice of Nursing Research: Appraisal, Synthesis, and Generation of Evidence. sixth ed. Saunders, St Louis.

Byrom, S., Downe, S., 2010. 'She sort of shines': midwives' accounts of 'good' midwifery and 'good' leadership. Midwifery 26 (1), 126–137.

Hindley, C., Hinsliff, S., Thomson, A., 2008. Pregnant womens' views about choice of intrapartum monitoring of the fetal heart rate: A questionnaire survey. Int. J. Nurs. Stud. 45 (2), 224–231.

Holloway, I., Wheeler, S., 2010. Qualitative Research in Nursing and Healthcare. third ed. Wiley-Blackwell, Chichester.

Houser, J., 2008. Nursing Research: Reading, Using and Creating Evidence. Jones and Bartlett, Boston.

Jackson, K., Fraser, D., 2009. A study exploring UK midwives' knowledge and attitudes towards caring for women who have been sexually abused. Midwifery 25 (3), 253–263.

Lacey, A., 2010. The research process. In: Gerrish, K., Lacey, A. (Eds.), The Research Process in Nursing, sixth ed. Wiley-Blackwell, Chichester.

McKeller, L., Pincombe, J., Henderson, A., 2008. Enhancing fathers' educational experiences during the early postnatal period. J. Perinat. Educ. 17 (4), 12–20.

Meyer, J., 2010. Action research. In: Gerrish, K., Lacey, A. (Eds.), The Research Process in Nursing, sixth ed. Wiley-Blackwell, Chichester.

Polit, D., Beck, C., 2008. Nursing Research: Generating and Assessing Evidence for Nursing Practice, eighth ed. Lippincott Williams and Wilkins, Philadelphia.

Punch, K., 2006. Developing Effective Research Proposals, second ed. Sage, London.

Schmidt, N., Brown, J., 2009. Evidence-Based Practice for Nurses: Appraisal and Application of Research. Jones and Bartlett, Boston.

Waterman, H., Hope, K., 2008. Action research. In: Watson, R., McKenna, H., Cowman, S., Keady, J. (Eds.), Nursing Research: Designs and Methods. Edinburgh, Churchill Livingstone.

Wood, M., Ross-Kerr, J., 2006. Basic Steps in Planning Nursing Research: From Question to Proposal, sixth ed. Jones and Bartlett, Boston.

Qualitative research approaches

4

Research comes in many shapes, sizes and 'brands'. As indicated in Chapter 2, one common broad categorisation is the distinction between *quantitative* and *qualitative* **research approaches. These terms are associated with the types of data produced by each category; however, a more fundamental difference is the researcher's beliefs concerning the nature of research, and the principles they should follow in completing it.**

As the majority of research used in evidence-based practice is quantitative, the aim of this chapter is to provide a balance between these two approaches by concentrating on qualitative research. It will extend the discussion on these two approaches in Chapter 2 by examining some of the main differences between quantitative and qualitative research, and describe three major types of qualitative designs. The importance of feminist approaches to midwifery will also be emphasised and its relationship to qualitative approaches outlined.

The development of health care knowledge has traditionally been associated with the 'scientific' image of research. This is particularly true of research used in evidence-based practice, which has focused largely on quantitative research, frequently in the form of randomised control trials (RCTs). This leaves qualitative research with many challenges, as it has not developed a similar strong position in health service decision making. In the past, the distinction between 'hard' and 'soft' data, and talk of a quantitative/qualitative 'divide' has exacerbated the view that qualitative research is in some way inferior to quantitative. Mauk (2009), for instance, points out that as a result of the principles of evidence-based practice, qualitative research is considered to be far less compelling than quantitative, which is seen as more objective methods and therefore 'sound'.

In reality, it is far better to see these as two distinct research approaches or 'research paradigms'. A *paradigm*, as we saw in Chapter 2, is a view and set of principles about the nature of something, like research, that shapes how people see and understand things related to that concept. In research, it influences the different ways researches who adopt either a quantitative or qualitative paradigm see the nature of research, its purpose and the role of the researcher.

© 2011 Elsevier Ltd. All rights reserved.

Each research paradigm can be seen to answer different types of questions; with both having an equal part to play in developing midwifery knowledge and practice. This is emphasised by Roberts and DiCenso (2008) who point out that no one research approach has precedent over another; it is the research question that should dictate the approach chosen. Particularly in midwifery, there are so many questions where best practice can be informed by research that focuses on understandings, interpretations and experiences, and which are more appropriate to a qualitative approach.

How does qualitative research differ from quantitative? The key difference is that qualitative research does not concentrate on the measurement of clinical outcomes; instead, it explores human experiences and processes, including those of midwives, and our understanding of health and illness issues from the perspective of those involved. Examples include women's experiences of Caesarian section (Fenwick et al. 2009) and midwives' interpretation of 'good' leadership and 'good' midwifery (Byrom and Downe 2010). Is this knowledge important to us? How can it not be? We need to understand how people experience health care if we are to provide a meaningful, sensitive and appropriate response to health needs. Pregnancy, birth and childcare are all extremely personal experiences, so any research approach that values human experience will be compatible with a profession that emphasises individuality, and an empowering approach to care. Qualitative research, then, is an appropriate choice in exploring some of the important issues facing midwifery.

The conclusion to be drawn from this is that all midwives need to be familiar with both quantitative and qualitative approaches to research if they are to demonstrate evidence-based practice. Qualitative approaches balance the narrow focus of quantitative research by examining the bigger picture, and the more human side of service provision. According to Houser (2008), it does have an important role to play in evidence-based practice, as it helps to determine the needs, preferences and motives of those receiving health care. The following section examines some of the major differences between the two major approaches of quantitative and qualitative methods.

THE CONTRAST BETWEEN QUANTITATIVE AND QUALITATIVE RESEARCH

Qualitative research is a broad term covering a number of different but related approaches to research. Burns and Grove (2009: 51) provide the following helpful description of it:

> *Qualitative research is a systematic, subjective approach used to describe life experiences and give them significance. It is a way to gain insights through discovering meanings. These insights are obtained not through establishing causality but through improving our comprehension of the whole.*

This emphasises that, like quantitative research, it is carried out in an organised and methodical way, but it contrasts with quantitative approaches in that its subject matter is human experiences, particularly the way in which people make sense of the things that happen to them. For this reason, qualitative research is sometimes referred to as *'constructivist research'*, as it is based on the belief that how we see things 'constructs' how we experience our reality or world, and these interpretations give it meaning (Houser 2008). Researchers using this approach try to identify these ways of constructing reality from the things that people say and do. Polit and Beck (2008) elaborate on this by outlining some of the key characteristics of qualitative approaches (see Box 4.1).

As these characteristics are important in understanding the differences between quantitative and qualitative research, they require further elaboration, as their meaning is not always clear. One way of simplifying matters is by demonstrating how the two approaches differ in the following three phases:

- planning,
- data collection, including role of the researcher and the nature of the relationship with those involved,
- analysis and interpretation of the results.

PLANNING

Perhaps the most important characteristic of qualitative research is the holistic approach that attempts to provide a total picture of individuals or group and their life experiences and beliefs. This is in contrast to isolating a single biophysical entity such as heart rate or blood pressure. This holistic approach of qualitative research is necessary if it is to discover how people interpret life events and give them meaning within their life. To achieve this, the researcher's exploration takes into account a broad outline of people's lives and cultural influences that may affect behaviour and beliefs and so allow the researcher to contextualise the topic and their findings (Holloway and Wheeler 2010). As a consequence, the research question will be broader than that found in quantitative research so that it can capture the bigger picture. The research process followed in qualitative research is also less structured and more flexible to adapt to new ideas and insights as they grow and develop throughout the study.

These features have considerable implications for the planning process, which tends to be shorter than in quantitative research. For example, less time is devoted to a comprehensive literature review. In the past, some qualitative

---

BOX 4.1 Characteristics of qualitative approaches to research

Qualitative design:
Often involves a merging together of various data collection strategies (i.e. triangulation);
Is flexible and elastic, capable of adjusting to what is being learned during the course of data collection;
Tends to be holistic, striving for an understanding of the whole;
Requires the researcher to become intensely involved, usually remaining in the field for lengthy periods of time;
Requires the researcher to become the research instrument; and
Requires ongoing analysis of the data to formulate subsequent strategies and to determine when fieldwork is done.

Polit and Beck 2008: 219.

researchers avoided a literature review in case it led to the analysis being 'contaminated' by previous research knowledge. However, this is less often followed now as the researcher should ensure the study has not already been undertaken, and consulting the literature will provide a broad understanding of concepts that may be related to the study (Holloway and Wheeler 2010). However, the literature should not 'direct' or 'influence' the path of the research. In qualitative research, the literature is used as part of data analysis where it is used as a way of confirming the credibility of the researcher's interpretations and descriptions of behaviour. This information will appear along with the data in the findings section. In contrast, quantitative studies do not include the literature in the results section, although it will appear in the discussion section.

A further planning stage distinction is that the qualitative researcher does not develop a structured tool of data collection based on the literature review, or use a tool that has been validated in previous research. This is because the researcher attempts to keep an open mind on what may be important within the study. The implication of this is that it is not possible to carry out a pilot study in the same way as in quantitative research, as there is no highly structured research tool to test for consistency and accuracy. Each interview or period of observation will be different and not standardised as in quantitative research, which seeks to ensure consistency.

DATA COLLECTION

In this phase of the research, the researcher may use more than one method of data collection to examine the concept of interest in the process of *triangulation*. Triangulation can include different research approaches or samples; here the term is used to describe the use of more than one tool of data collection in a study. Triangulation is a common feature of qualitative research where it is used to consolidate or confirm the picture emerging from one tool of data collection.

One of the clearest differences between the two research approaches is the way the researcher forms a relationship with the sample during data collection. As the aim of the research is to gain an understanding and insight into human behaviour, there is a social closeness in the relationship between the researcher and the participants. This mainly develops over a sustained time period not characterised by the quick interview or the faceless questionnaire approach. Traditionally, in quantitative research there is a belief that the researcher should keep a social distance from the subjects of the research to avoid undue influence on the results. Although the quantitative researcher supports the idea of maintaining a 'rapport' with subjects, this does not relate to the same level of intimacy and closeness evident in many examples of qualitative research. This takes on a particular significance where both the researcher and participants are female. The more intimate, flexible, and more reciprocal the relationship between both parties in qualitative research is in harmony with the philosophy of feminist research, the more there is an attempt to minimise any inequalities in power between the researcher and participants. This balance in the relationship is crucial in feminist research, which aims to give women's experiences a voice and where the goal of the research is to empower women (Holloway and Wheeler 2010).

This means that the researcher must have a great deal of personal awareness of the relationship with subjects where this may have influenced the findings. This is referred to as *reflexivity*, where the researcher considers the extent to which he or she may have shaped the findings as part of the process of data collection (Houser 2008). The impact of the researcher on data gathering has led commentators such as Holloway and Wheeler (2010) to describe the researcher in qualitative research as the tool of data collection or research instrument, in that the researcher makes decisions on what should be regarded as data and what should be highlighted through the analysis and presentation of findings.

DATA ANALYSIS AND INTERPRETATION

Visually, one of the clearest differences between quantitative and qualitative research is the form of data presentation; the former is presented using numbers and analysed statistically, and the latter using words in the form of direct quotations and descriptions of activities and is analysed through the researcher's interpretation of emerging themes, although computer software can also be used as part of this process.

The sequence of events between data gathering and analysis is also different. Unlike quantitative research where the process of analysis starts once data collection has finished, in qualitative research data gathering and data analysis are carried out at the same time. Fieldwork may stop when the researcher feels that no new themes or elements are emerging and 'data saturation' has been reached, that is, when further data collection would be redundant.

Analysis in qualitative research is characterised by an *inductive* approach rather than a *deductive* one. This means that the researcher takes the individual elements emerging from the analysis and gradually builds up a picture to provide a broad explanation of what may be happening. In contrast, the quantitative researcher starts with general principles, often in the form of a theory or hypothesis, and examines the individual units of data to either confirm or reject that theory or hypothesis.

It is not an exaggeration then, to say that in so many aspects of the research process, the two approaches of quantitative and qualitative are worlds apart. This is illustrated in Table 4.1, which illustrates some of the major differences. The following section examines some of the more popular qualitative approaches to illustrate the qualitative approach further.

QUALITATIVE RESEARCH DESIGNS

Although qualitative research can take many different forms, there are three main categories or 'traditions' (Houser 2008) that dominate nursing and midwifery research, all of which seek an '*emic*' or insider view of a particular topic or situation. This is in contrast to the '*etic*' or researcher and outsider's viewpoint. The three main methods are:

- ethnography,
- phenomenology,
- grounded theory.

Each of these will now be considered.

Table 4.1 *Summary of differences between quantitative and qualitative approaches*

Characteristic	Quantitative	Qualitative
Focus	Narrow and specific	Holistic and general
Research question	Precisely worded	Broadly worded
Type of evidence	Objective	Subjective
Belief about reality and research activity	The social world is similar to other 'sciences' and open to measurement by the researcher. Reality is 'out there' and objective	The social world can only be known through an individual's experience and understanding of it. Reality is inside all of us
Researcher's relationship to subjects	Detached to ensure it does not influence subjects, although rapport sought	More equal and reciprocal relationship characterised by social warmth
Review of the literature	Critical to the development of the process	Can be used to provide a broad picture, but often used to support findings. It is included as part of written report.
Planning	Carried out in depth	High level of planning avoided so as to reduce preconceived ideas about the nature of the topic
Tool of data collection	Emphasis on accuracy and consistency, to ensure reliability and validity	As the tool is used flexibly and continually developing, it is impossible to pilot to determine consistency and accuracy
Sample size	Emphasis on large numbers to reduce bias and to allow statistical procedures	Small numbers but appropriate experience explored
Sample referred to as	Subjects	'Informants' or 'participants' to avoid dehumanising
Analytical approach	Deductive	Inductive
Data	Numeric	Words
Data gathering	Extensive to gain maximum coverage	Intensive to gain maximum depth and rich, 'thick' data
Product of data analysis	Referred to as 'results'	Referred to as 'findings', although some publications use the term 'results'
Generalisability	Major concern to achieve this to a high level	Not a major concern, low level achieved
Ethical concerns	High, particularly where an intervention is invasive	High, harm is concerned with psychological and social elements and the protection of human dignity

Table 4.1 *Summary of differences between quantitative and qualitative approaches—Cont'd*

Characteristic	Quantitative	Qualitative
Methodological concerns	Reliability, validity and bias	Trustworthiness, in the form of credibility, dependability, confirmability and transferability
Emphasis on rigour	High	High
Application to evidence-based practice	Highly rated, notably in the form of RCTs	Presently low acceptability, increasing emphasis on user views and experiences may change this
Applicability to midwifery practice	High	High

ETHNOGRAPHY

The holistic approach taken by the qualitative researcher is clearly illustrated in the work of the ethnographer. Burns and Grove (2009: 57) characterise ethnography as producing a 'portrait of a people', while Holloway and Wheeler (2010: 153) describe it as a way of 'studying human behaviour in the context of a culture in order to gain understanding of cultural rules, norms and routines'. It is not surprising then, to find that this approach has its roots in anthropology, where the objective of the anthropologist was to describe and interpret human activities within a culture or cultural subgroup. These were usually pre-literature and 'exotic' groups or tribes where the researcher attempted to learn something about the people and the society as a whole.

Rather than choosing exotic and 'non-literate' tribes, the use of this approach is now applied to everyday cultures, but still with the purpose of understanding the rituals and beliefs that people hold and that influence their behaviour. The underlying assumption of ethnographic research, according to Polit and Beck (2008: 224) is that every human group evolves a culture that guides the members' view of the world and the way they structure their experiences. The aim of the ethnographer is to learn from (rather than to study as in a laboratory) members of a cultural group. This again gives clues as to the way qualitative researchers think and the values they hold about research.

The anthropologist's techniques of observation, interviews, participation and immersion in the culture, have all been adopted to various extents by the ethnographic researcher in health care. Like the original anthropologists, the ethnographer is described as carrying out *'fieldwork'*, that is, a study in the natural environment or 'field' in which those involved in the study are usually found. This usually lasts for sustained periods of time in order to observe a particular group under a range of circumstances. This does hold dangers, as the longer the period of observation, the more likely a close and familiar relationship develops between the observer and the observed. This can lead to what anthropologists call *'going native'*. This means the researcher no longer sees the group's activities through the eyes of an enquiring stranger, but rather as another member of the group with 'taken for granted' or 'tacit' knowledge. To overcome this, the researcher attempts to use the technique of *'cultural strangeness'*. This means trying to see things 'with the eye of an outsider' (Holloway and Wheeler 2010), so that they can question the purpose and meaning of behaviour those within the group see as unremarkable. This is perhaps one of the difficulties facing the midwife ethnographer, in that it is very difficult to see things as culturally strange once socialised into the midwifery role.

There are also practical difficulties facing the midwife ethnographer, particularly the investment of sufficient time to carry out the fieldwork. Polit and Beck (2008: 225) refer to ethnographic research as a typically labour-intensive and time-consuming endeavour. This is because the researcher first needs time to gain trust and acceptance, and a clearly identified role within the group. It is a very intimate relationship where those in the study are prepared to share deep feelings and shared understandings that they may not want to reveal to strangers. This makes for a potentially expensive study in terms of time required.

Anthropologists are typically concerned with what people do and say, and how it is said, the objects they make or use and how they use them. This helps us understand the approach of such studies and the focus of attention. The methods of data collection to achieve these aims typically consist of observation and interviews, both of which tend to be flexible and intense, that is, they are carried out over a long period of time in the field. Other forms of data collection can also be used to shed light on the situation such as written accounts, including health records or diaries. The approach of ethnography is very similar to making a 'fly-on-the-wall' documentary. The purpose is not to manipulate a situation, but rather record it and try and make sense of it. Instead of a camera, ethnographic researchers keep a 'fieldwork diary' in which they capture the details of their observations, interviews and their personal interpretations and understandings. In presenting results, reference may be made to a fieldwork diary or field notes to add detail and support the accuracy of the observations and interviews.

One illustration of this is the work of Crozier et al. (2007), who set out to explore midwifery competence in the use of birth technology, including such equipment as electronic fetal monitoring (EFM) syringe drivers, infusion pumps, monitors and computers. The lead researcher shadowed 16 midwives in the cultural setting of two hospitals providing a mix of midwife-led and consultant-led care. The data were collected through detailed participant observation and conversation with midwives. The observations and conversations were recorded as field notes and analysed for common themes. The study concluded that midwives showed competence and confidence in the use of birth technologies but the findings did raise some issues for education in regard to the midwives' interpretations of readings produced by these technologies.

PHENOMENOLOGY

Although it is relatively easy to summarise the broad purpose of phenomenology, the ideas underpinning this approach are very complex and will be simplified considerably here to provide a general view of its features. Some of the complexity of the approach stems from its origins in the discipline of philosophy. It attempts to understand the essential nature of people's experiences and interpretations of key features in their life so that the core *essence* of a concept can be revealed. 'Essence', according to Polit and Beck (2008: 227), is *'what makes a phenomenon what it is, and without which it would not be what it is'*.

This is clearly useful for the midwifery researcher who wants to understand the essence of the experiences that women encounter during pregnancy, birth and motherhood, so that the experiences can be understood by midwives.

As with other qualitative approaches, there is not one 'method' that produces a phenomenological study, but several variations. Many researchers who claim to follow this approach credit the influence of one of two key German philosophers, Edmund Husserl (1859–1938), and one of his students, Martin Heidegger (1889–1976) who developed Husserl's ideas in a different direction. However, the philosophy of phenomenology has also been influenced by French thinkers, such as Maurice Merleau-Ponty (1908–1961) and Paul Ricoeur (1913–2005). These influential figures were not researchers, but their philosophical ideas have influenced the way that phenomenological researchers think about the purpose of their research and how people experience the world. As a research method, phenomenology can be defined as a method of gaining the lived experience of a particular phenomenon as seen through the eyes of those involved so that its essence can be discovered. The phrase *'lived experience'* is often found in the title of such studies.

Phenomenological research is typically conducted by means of in-depth interviews. The approach will differ depending on whose work has influenced the study. For example, if the main influence comes from Husserl, the emphasis will be on a descriptive approach to the lived experience. Here, the researcher is encouraged to put aside one's personal understandings, values and preconceptions. This is attempted through the process of *'bracketing'* where the researcher's views are put on one side so as not to influence data collection and interpretation. Those following Heidegger do not attempt to bracket; and the focus is on the interpretation of what it is like for those in the study, and where prior understanding of the topic or situation is a necessary part of the researcher's interpretation. A great deal of controversy exists in the literature over the process of bracketing, particularly in regard to whether it is possible to suspend what we already know (Gelling 2010), and what the researcher should do when attempting to 'bracket' (Hamill and Sinclair 2010).

Phenomenology has a great deal to offer midwifery, as it provides the perspective of those receiving services and so might open up understandings that may not be available through other methods. One example of this approach is the work by Dibley (2009), who undertook a study of 10 lesbian parents' experiences of health care in the UK, focusing on interactions with midwives. She adopted a Heideggerian phenomenological approach for the study as she wanted to use her own experiences as a lesbian mother and nurse to interpret the findings without 'bracketing' her own connectedness with the topic of the study. Thus it can be argued that the positive bias that this might have provided enhances the quality of the study. The study provides stark information on the way some lesbian mothers are treated by midwives and gives clear recommendations on improvements that need to be made to increase the quality of experience for this group of women.

GROUNDED THEORY

This is the most recent research approach and was developed in the 1960s by two American sociologists, Glaser and Strauss, to explore hospital staff's behaviour towards dying patients. Although the approach may look similar to either a phenomenological study or an ethnographic study, the crucial difference is in its purpose. Whereas the aim of the former approaches is to describe by painting a word picture of a situation or, as in the case of interpretative phenomenology, to add meaning and therefore arrive at understanding, the purpose of grounded theory is not only to describe but also to try to explain, through a proposition of why things might take the forms they do. These propositions can be said to form a theory that is 'grounded' in the data collected; hence the term 'grounded theory'. As with other forms of qualitative research, variations have grown out of its original form. This has led Parahoo (2009) to remark that no other qualitative research approach has spawned such a large volume of literature discussing its essential nature.

In grounded theory, data collection and analysis are carried out in parallel, and stop once 'saturation' occurs, that is, no more new analytical categories arise. The analysis also consists of *'the constant comparison method'* where new data and emerging categories from the analysis are compared with previous data and categories to ensure consistency and the possible development of links between the categories.

Grounded theory uses methods such as observation alone or with other methods, such as interviews. These are similar to the previous two qualitative approaches in being very flexible in design. An important source is also the fieldwork diary in which researchers keep a running commentary on the way events unfold and their own reflections and developing understanding of the situation. The main emphasis in the findings section of a grounded theory study is the presentation of a model or theory that explains the data collected. It is through these theoretical models that midwifery theory can be expanded and practice developed in line with the experiences and perceptions of both midwives and those for whom they care.

QUALITATIVE RESEARCH WITHIN MIDWIFERY

The previous sections have indicated how each approach or 'tradition' has been applied within midwifery, and some of these are illustrated in Table 4.2. However, as qualitative research takes so many diverse approaches, not all midwifery research falls neatly into one of these categories. Indeed, as can be seen from Table 4.2, researchers may simply state that they have broadly followed a quantitative approach and not specify a particular category. In these instances, they may have followed some of the basic principles of a qualitative approach in valuing the individual's views, experiences or perceptions, or have followed some of the principles of qualitative data analysis to make sense of the findings.

The depth of analysis will also vary from article to article. In some examples the researcher will use a more descriptive approach to present the study and summarise the main points made under various headings. Here, the attempt is to paint a picture of the situation from the individual's perspective without attempting to provide analytical comment. These articles can be of practical value, although they might not follow the criteria applied to the qualitative approaches described above. In other examples, the researcher may provide far more detailed analysis and provide more in-depth 'backstage' information on how the study was carried out and the analysis achieved.

Table 4.2 Examples of midwifery qualitative research

Author and year	Aim	Stated approach	Sample size	Sampling strategy	Tool(s) of data collection	Method of analysis
Fenwick et al. (2009)	To explore women's experiences of Caesarean section.	Grounded theory	21	Purposive	Interviews	Coding and categorising and constant comparison method
Fraser and Hughes (2009)	To explore the factors that influence student midwives' constructs of childbearing, before and during their undergraduate midwifery programme	This research followed an overall naturalistic methodology	58	Self-selecting volunteers	Focus Groups	Transcripts were entered into QSR NVivov7 (computer programme) and both members of the research team coded the data and analysed the emerging themes independently, before meeting to assess the findings.
Byrom and Downe (2010)	To explore midwives' accounts of the characteristics of 'good' leadership and 'good' midwifery.	Phenomenological	10	Random sampling stratified to encompass senior and junior grades	Interviews	Thematic analysis, carried out manually.
Crozier et al. (2007)	To explore midwifery competence in the use of birth technology.	Ethnographic	16	Purposive	Observation and 'conversations'	Coding and analysis of data took place with the use of NVivo software for qualitative analysis.
Keating and Fleming (2009)	To explore midwives' experiences of facilitating normal birth in an obstetric-led unit.	Feminist	10	Purposive	Interviews	Identification of themes using feminist theory (Warren's 4 concepts of patriarchy)

4 FEMINIST RESEARCH

Qualitative researchers will often state that they have drawn on a particular approach such as a phenomenology or grounded theory as a part of the methodology section of a research article. This helps the reader anticipate the way the material has been analysed and the thinking behind that analysis. In midwifery there are a surprisingly small number of studies that follow a *feminist research* tradition, despite the stated aim of midwifery being to be woman-centred. The reason for this underrepresentation is not clear.

The aim of this section is to consider what is meant by feminist research and its relevance to midwifery knowledge. The starting point is to place feminist research within the context of feminism. As a social movement, feminism takes many forms, but in essence, the ideals, of feminism relate to the following three areas:

- a valuing of, and emphasis on, the experiences, opinions, ideals and needs of women as a group in society,
- the oppression of women in society by a dominant culture of male power,
- a desire to improve the position of women in society and the quality of their lives.

Feminism is based on the belief that gender is a fundamental organiser of social life, according to writers such as Kelly et al. (1995). In other words, many of the things that happen (or do not happen) to women are because of the way in which males influence all aspects of life to the detriment and disadvantage of women. Men are held to dominate and dismiss the value of women and their views in all spheres of life, even to the extent that women become sidelined and 'invisible' in the leading decision-making arenas of social and organisational life. A major goal of feminism is to raise the profile of women and give them a legitimate voice by redressing the imbalance of power in society. A further goal is the acceptance and legitimisation of a female social agenda and the development of an action plan for the issues raised by it. This is accepted as a long struggle, as it is felt that the negative position of women in society has existed for so long that many women themselves no longer question the disadvantages they face and have come to see them as 'normal'.

Women's health can be seen as a particular area in which women are vulnerable and do not always have the power to control the process in which they are involved. Throughout the life cycle, women's reproductive and general health becomes controlled by medicine. The history of obstetric care is a good example of how a predominantly male obstetric profession has dominated the ideas and discussion on what constitutes a desirable form of care for women during pregnancy and birth. This has led to some clearly oppressive situations for women in the name of safety and convenience. The quality of the birth experience and subsequent relationship with their baby has also been influenced by obstetric values and practices. In all of this, midwifery can find itself supporting a situation that is part of women's powerlessness. This is illustrated by the feminist analysis of Keating and Fleming (2009) who identify the difficulties midwives face in trying to facilitate a normal birth in an obstetric-led unit in Ireland. The conclusions of this study of births in three units found that midwives were impeded in their attempts to support normal birth practices by the culture of the birth setting, and the hierarchy of health staff who supported a medical philosophy of birth.

Feminist research developed in response to the dissatisfaction felt by some researchers that the definition of research and the way it was conducted was overly influenced by the dominance of male researchers and a male approach to research, that is, distant and disengaged from those who were its 'subjects'. It was felt that the quantitative research agenda neglected many of the questions that would benefit women, and feminist research was developed to form a more appropriate approach to addressing issues that were seen as woman-centred and ignored by the current research agenda. It sought to ensure that the relationship between a female researcher and the women taking part in the study was not exploitative, but more equal and based on a sharing of information and knowledge. The methods used were mainly interviews but were more like conversations, with a greater social balance between the two individuals involved. Similarly, an attempt was made to ensure that the production of written or audio narratives were more under the control of the women themselves and highlighted their 'voice' on issues seen as important to them.

So, how do we define feminist research? Holloway and Wheeler (2010: 258) state that:

> *Feminist inquiry is research that focuses on the experiences, ideas and feelings of women in their social and historical context.... The intention is to make women visible, raise their consciousness and empower them.*

This definition clearly helps to identify the purpose of feminist research and the themes it highlights. Again, there are a number of different forms that feminist research can take, but all follow the principles of going further than just the generation of knowledge by contributing to the improvement of the position of women through greater social justice and social change (Kralik and van Loon 2008).

Unfortunately, this approach has not had a great impact on nursing and midwifery research. Indeed, earlier writers such as Sigsworth (1995) took great pains to point out the benefits of feminist research by stressing that it provides a more relevant way of thinking about, and carrying out research, in comparison to the more customary randomised control trial, yet, there seems to have been little response to such arguments.

One relatively recent exception is the work of Johnson et al. (2009), who examine how women's way of talking about expressing breast milk to feed their baby illustrates the pressure to be a good mother and still overcome real practical problems in breastfeeding, such as breastfeeding in public or overcoming pain when breastfeeding. Following the analysis of a larger study, 16 participants were identified as having expressed breast milk for a number of reasons. The analysis of audio diaries and interviews within a feminist framework suggested that expressing breast milk was used as a compromise to the pressure to conform to the principle of 'breast is best' and ensuring 'good' mothering, despite significant difficulties in breastfeeding itself. In this respect, the study emphasises the experiences of this group of women through the use of their own words and demonstrates ways of maintaining individual autonomy, although the authors identify that the findings can be interpreted in a number of different ways within a feminist framework.

This section emphasises the way in which research is not just simply a process that is totally objective, but a process that can make a statement concerning a group as a whole, such as women in society. Although the tools employed are similar to those used elsewhere, it is the philosophy or values underpinning the way the study was conducted and interpreted that holds the key. Here it is argued that feminist research has much to offer midwifery research, and that at the moment it is grossly underutilised as a legitimate methodology within the profession.

CONDUCTING RESEARCH

Once the researcher has decided that a qualitative or 'interpretative' approach is appropriate, a particular category of qualitative method has to be selected. The wording of the research question and purposes of the research will provide some guidance. Questions that ask 'what it is like to have a certain experience, such as elective Caesarean section, or twins', may require more of a phenomenological approach that uncovers the 'lived experience' of individuals. If the question is concerned with behaviour or the structure of activities of an identified group or 'culture', such as midwives or breastfeeding women, then a more ethnographic approach will be appropriate. If the approach sets out to provide an explanation for a particular activity or belief, such as why do some women feel that birth in a midwifery-led unit is the preferred option, then a grounded theory approach should be adopted.

Although these different qualitative forms of research originally followed strict principles, through use and changing ideas, variations and adaptations have arisen. The flexibility of these approaches has sometimes made it difficult to find consensual guidelines for those wanting to carry out this type of research. There is also a lack of learning opportunities to study and practice the techniques of data collection and analysis required by these approaches. For this reason, this type of research is more usually 'informed by' a particular approach or tradition rather than following it to the letter.

In the same way that quantitative researchers must ensure that they fully understand the process of quantitative data collection and analysis, so qualitative researchers must ensure that their work is carried out ethically and rigorously. A number of helpful texts now exist that provide some guidance on the conduct of qualitative research (Silverman 2010, Holloway and Wheeler 2010), and how it should be written up (Wolcott 2009). It is advised that potential qualitative researchers study these texts, and participate in courses that specialise in this form of research. The novice qualitative researcher should also read as many examples of this type of research as possible in order to get a feel for the way it is conducted and presented.

This is not an easy choice of approach, particularly with phenomenology, because of its history and underpinning with philosophy. Where possible, try to read articles that describe the researcher's experiences in conducting qualitative research. Hunt and Symond's (1995) work remains a classic and very readable account of a qualitative study that includes many 'backstage' details.

The book describes in great detail many of the problems, pitfalls and dilemmas Hunt encountered in carrying out her research in a midwifery unit. Similarly, there are a number of nursing researchers who have also written 'behind-the-scene' accounts of their experiences as a novice researcher undertaking qualitative research. For example, Vivar (2007) provides advice on writing a qualitative research proposal; Skene (2007) and Bailey (2007) both provide their experience of undertaking qualitative research; Simmons (2007) shares her experience of phenomenological research, while Wilson (2008) describes her experience of grounded theory. All of these provide important pointers for the qualitative researcher.

Ethical considerations are just as important with this type of research as with quantitative approaches. One added difficulty, however, is that ethics committees may not be totally familiar with the approach of qualitative research in comparison to quantitative approaches. Some researchers have, therefore, found it useful to attach brief extracts or explanations of techniques or procedures from research texts as part of a submission. Contacting the ethics committee in advance to ask whether to include this kind of detail is a further option.

In carrying out qualitative research, one ethical dilemma is the emotional closeness established between midwifery researcher and participant. This can lead to details of behaviour or descriptions of events being revealed that might oblige the researcher to break the confidentiality between the researcher and participant. An example might be a confession regarding conduct towards a child that might suggest the child is at risk. Under the professional code of conduct, a midwifery researcher would have to report that confession or detail. When outlining the nature of the researcher's role, participants should be told that if certain information is revealed to them, the researcher might have an obligation to inform others. Similarly, if participants seem close to revealing information that might lead to this, they should be reminded of the researcher's duty to break confidences.

It should also be remembered that the nature of qualitative research is very intensive and emotionally challenging. Support from supervisors and personal support can be important in managing the emotional demands that arise.

Finally, if the research question relates to the disadvantage of women during this vulnerable period of their life or highlights the disadvantages faced by women in general, and the intention is to highlight and possibly reduce this problem, then a feminist approach is relevant.

CRITIQUING RESEARCH

As qualitative research is so different from quantitative research, the same approach to critiquing cannot be used. More details of this will be given in the next chapter on critiquing.

The first stage is to confirm that a study is qualitative in nature and then to identify which type of approach has been used. Although articles will usually indicate their qualitative nature in the title, or at least in the methods section, some authors go no further than stating that their research is qualitative in nature. This means that the method of critiquing can only be broad, and the specific criteria associated with the various approaches cannot be used. However, it is important to satisfy yourself that the common elements that unite qualitative approaches are present.

As with quantitative research, the important question in reading qualitative research is, 'can I trust it'. In quantitative research, the key concepts are reliability and validity. It is also important to establish if the research is generalisable. As we shall see in the next chapter, in qualitative research the emphasis is different, as the methods of undertaking research follow different principles. The relevant concepts include *credibility*, *auditability* and *fittingness*.

Credibility is concerned with the trustworthiness of the findings. Are they accurate descriptions of what was said or done? This is sometimes confirmed either by checking written accounts with those who participated in the research that they are a true record of the interview or observation; this is called a *'member's check'*. Alternatively, or sometimes in addition, the researcher checks with peers to establish whether others would come to the same conclusions or categories.

Auditability is concerned with the extent to which the researcher illustrates the progress from individual comments or observations to themes. It illustrates how researchers developed their analysis to show that it is based on an inductive process. Usually, in the methods section there will be details on the procedure followed to analyse the findings. This may have the name of someone's approach to analysis such as van Manen, Giorgi, or Colaizzi, all of whom are regularly used as guides to data analysis.

Fittingness is concerned with the extent to which the basic principles can be applied to other situations, much as in quantitative research where there is an attempt to illustrate the generalisability of the results.

Although many people find statistical presentations of results in quantitative research intimidating, the unfamiliar terminology and thinking behind qualitative research can also be challenging. As qualitative research has a great deal to offer midwifery knowledge, do not be inhibited by unfamiliar terminology or ideas; instead, try to identify the underlying messages that can be applied to practice. You should find that qualitative research can be more engaging and interesting than the presentation of many quantitative studies because of its emphasis on the spoken words and feelings of those caught up in midwifery care.

KEY POINTS

- Although quantitative research has a long history as the 'brand leader' in health care research, qualitative and quantitative research approaches do different jobs and answer different types of questions.
- Qualitative research is concerned with illuminating the interpretations and meanings people give to features in their life, including those relating to pregnancy, birth and parenthood. This leads to a more holistic and person-centred approach to generating knowledge than does quantitative research.
- Three major categories or traditions within qualitative research are ethnographic, phenomenological and grounded theory. However, many other different approaches exist. All have in common an attempt to present situations through the eyes of those involved. This means that researchers must try to avoid enforcing their preconceived ideas on the processes of data collection and

analysis. The issues and themes should emerge from the data collected and be directed and controlled as much as possible by those supplying those insights.
- Qualitative research is frequently characterised by a close relationship between the researcher and those participating in the study. Indeed, to a very large extent the researcher is the tool of data collection in qualitative research whose social skills are paramount to effective data collection.
- Issues relating to rigour and ethical considerations are just as important in this type of research as in quantitative research.
- Feminist approaches to research contain many of the characteristics of qualitative methods. Feminist research seeks to improve the situation of women disadvantaged by their position as women within health care arenas.
- It is easy for some people to dismiss qualitative research if they have used criteria only relevant to critiquing quantitative research. Knowledge of the principles of qualitative research is fundamental to an accurate critique of such studies.
- Midwives need an understanding of both types of research in order to take a balanced approach to evidence-based practice.

REFERENCES

Bailey, C., 2007. Practitioner to researcher: reflections on the journey. Nurse Res. 14 (4), 18–26.

Burns, N., Grove, S., 2009. The Practice of Nursing Research: Appraisal, Synthesis, and Generation of Evidence, sixth ed. Saunders, St Louis.

Byrom, S., Downe, S., 2010. 'She sort of shines': midwives' accounts of 'good' midwifery and 'good' leadership. Midwifery 26 (1), 126–137.

Crozier, K., Sinclair, M., Kernohan, W., Porter, S., 2007. Ethnography of technological competence in clinical midwifery practice. Evidence Based Midwifery 5 (2), 59–65.

Dibley, L., 2009. Experiences of lesbian parents in the UK: interactions with midwives. Evidence Based Midwifery 7 (3), 94–100.

Fenwick, S., Holloway, I., Alexander, J., 2009. Achieving normality: The key to status passage to motherhood after a caesarean section. Midwifery 25 (5), 554–563.

Fraser, D., Hughes, A., 2009. Perceptions of motherhood: The effect of experience and knowledge on midwifery students. Midwifery 25 (3), 307–316.

Gelling, L., 2010. Phenomenology: the methodological minefield. Nurse Res. 17 (2), 4–6.

Hamill, C., Sinclair, H., 2010. Bracketing – practical considerations in Husserlian phenomenological research. Nurse Res. 17 (2), 16–24.

Holloway, I., Wheeler, S., 2010. Qualitative Research for Nurses, third ed. Wiley-Blackwell, Chichester.

Houser, J., 2008. Nursing Research: Reading, Using and Creating Evidence. Jones and Bartlett, Sudbury.

Hunt, S., Symonds, A., 1995. The Social Meaning of Midwifery. Macmillan, Houndmills.

Johnson, S., Williamson, I., Lyttle, S., Leeming, D., 2009. Expressing yourself: A feminist analysis of talk around expressing breast milk. Soc. Sci. Med. 69 (6), 900–907.

Keating, A., Fleming, V., 2009. Midwives' experiences of facilitating normal birth in an obstetric-led unit: a feminist perspective. Midwifery 25 (5), 518–527.

Kelly, L., Regan, L., Burton, S., 1995. Defending the indefensible? Quantitative methods and feminist research. In: Holland, J., Blair, M., Sheldon, S. (Eds.), Debates and Issues in Feminist research and Pedagogy. Multilingual Matters Ltd. In association with The Open University, Clevedon.

Kralik, D., van Loon, A., 2008. Feminist research. In: Watson, R., McKenna, H., Cowman, S., Keady, J. (Eds.), Nursing Research: Designs and Methods. Churchill Livingstone, Edinburgh.

Mauk, K., 2009. Qualitative designs: Using words to produce evidence. In: Schmidt, N., Brown, J. (Eds.), Evidence-Based Practice for Nurses. Jones and Bartlett, Sudbury.

Parahoo, K., 2009. Grounded theory: what's the point. Nurse Res. 17 (1), 4–7.

Polit, D., Beck, C., 2008. Nursing Research: Generating and Assessing Evidence for Nursing Practice, eighth ed. Lippincott Williams and Wilkins, Philadelphia.

Roberts, J., DiCenso, A., 2008. Identifying the best research design to fit the question. Part 1: quantitative research. In: Cullum, N., Ciliska, D., Haynes, R., Marks, S. (Eds.), Evidence-Based Nursing: An Introduction. Blackwell, Oxford.

Sigsworth, J., 1995. Feminist research: its relevance to nursing. J. Adv. Nurs. 22, 896–899.

Silverman, D., 2010. Doing Qualitative Research, third ed. Sage, London.

Simmons, M., 2007. Insider ethnography: tinker, tailor, researcher or spy? Nurse Res 14 (4), 7–17.

Skene, C., 2007. Interviewing women: using reflection to improve practice. Nurse Res 14 (4), 53–63.

Vivar, C., 2007. Getting started with qualitative research: developing a research proposal. Nurse Res 14 (3), 60–73.

Wilson, M., 2008. Snakes and ladders: reflections of a novice researcher. Nurse Res 15 (3), 4–11.

Wolcott, H., 2009. Writing Up Qualitative Research, third ed. Sage, Thousand Oaks.

Critiquing research articles 5

The main purpose of midwifery research is to increase the quality of care through the application of evidence-based knowledge gained from systematic data collection and analysis. There is a problem, however, and that is research does vary in quality. The perfect research project is almost impossible to achieve as researchers seldom have ideal conditions in which to carry out their work and so find themselves making the best of a bad job. So how does the midwife reading research distinguish between the good, the misleading and the dangerous? Developing critiquing skills is part of the answer. This chapter clarifies the meaning and purpose of critiquing. The skill of critiquing is illustrated with the aid of two critiquing frameworks; one for qualitative research articles and the other for qualitative research. Some of the details within both frameworks are based on information in later chapters. This means that you may need to look at these for more details on certain points. This chapter appears at this point in the book as critiquing is a skill that should be developed early in gaining an understanding of research.

Some research skills all midwives need to develop, and critiquing is one of them. This is because, as Lavender (2010) emphasises, it is no good relying on others to critique research for you as they may have a different agenda and interpret studies differently. You must be able to do this for yourself. According to Burns and Grove (2009: 598), critiquing, or critical appraisal, means the systematic, unbiased careful examination of all aspects of a study in order to judge the merits, limitations, meaning and relevance to practice. Although the word critique sounds like the word 'criticise', it is meant to be a constructive evaluation, and should be objective, unbiased and impartial. It should take a balanced view of both the content and process of research as followed by an author. It is a way of using critical skills to reflect on not only the whole process in which the research was undertaken, but also the thinking and assumptions on which the research was based.

Critiquing is a skill that requires practice, so read this chapter with a research article that is not too complex by your side. This will help you become familiar with applying the critique framework. In the first section you will need a

© 2011 Elsevier Ltd. All rights reserved.

quantitative study, where the results are presented in the form of numbers, and in the second part, a qualitative study where dialogue, quotes or descriptions of events are used.

APPLYING A CRITIQUING FRAMEWORK

Before starting to critique it is useful to consider the words of McCarthy and O'Sullivan (2008), who suggest that as time is so short and so much evidence available, we should firstly consider if an individual paper is worth reading. How do we tell? The first of two criteria that will help is to limit your effort to peer-reviewed articles. This will indicate it is from a reliable source, such as a well-known professional journal that first gets experts to check that the study is worthy of publication. Secondly, consider the title and its relevance to the topic you are exploring. Once you have chosen your article, there are three questions that need to be answered:

- What does it say?
- Can I trust it?
- Will it contribute to practice?

The first question relates to comprehension and is a description of what the authors examined. How did they justify the need for the study? How did they carry out the study? What did they find? What did they conclude? The second question relates to an assessment of the rigour applied to the research process – how well was it thought through, and what steps were taken to reduce problems of bias, reliability and validity. This second question requires knowledge of some of the kinds of issues and techniques of research covered throughout this book. The third question relates to an evaluation of the study's contribution to professional practice – does it provide clear evidence for continuing, adapting or challenging practice. Who might benefit from the study, and in what way?

Starting with the question of comprehension and what the research says, we might feel that if we read through an article we will know what it says. This is not necessarily the case. For instance, have you ever started reading at the top of a page, but by the time you have reached the bottom you have no recollection of what you have just read at the top? This is because most of us read passively a great deal of the time. Reading research articles is very different from reading a novel as they require a far more active, analytical and reflective approach.

To help us improve our active reading and analytical skills we need two things; first of all, we need to separate a research article into its component parts. This will allow us to see the overall outline of the research, and understand how all the pieces fit together. Secondly, to be an active reader we need questions to which we actively seek answers. Box 5.1 provides such a framework and a list of questions for quantitative research articles. The following sections will add detail to the framework.

FOCUS

The first thing we need to identify is the broad topic the research covers, so we can put it in the context of existing knowledge. This should be stated in a few words that include the key concepts or variables covered in the article.

BOX 5.1 Framework for critiquing quantitative research

You should not expect to get answers to every question in each section, as what is important will vary from study to study. The questions provided here are to give you some guidance.

1. Focus

   In broad terms, what is the theme of the article? What are the key words you would file this under? Is the title a clue to the focus? How important is this for the profession/practice?

2. Background

   What argument or evidence does the researcher provide to suggest this topic is worth exploring? Is there a review of previous literature on the subject, or reference to government or professional reports that illustrate its importance? Are gaps in the literature or inadequacies with previous methods highlighted? Are local problems or changes that justify the study presented? Is there a trigger that answers the question, 'why did they do it then'? Is there a theoretical or conceptual framework that helps us to see how all the elements in the study may be related?

3. Aim

   What is the aim of the research? This will usually start with the word 'to', e.g. the aim of this research was 'to examine/determine/compare/establish/etc'. If relevant, is there a hypothesis? If there is, what are the dependent and independent variables? Are there concept and operational definitions for the key concepts?

4. Study design

   What is the broad research approach? Is it quantitative or qualitative? Is the design experimental, descriptive or correlation? Is the study design appropriate to the aim?

5. Data collection method

   Which tool of data collection has been used? Has a single method been used or triangulation? Has the author addressed the issues of reliability and validity? Has a pilot study been conducted or tool used from previous studies? Have any limitations of the tool been recognised?

6. Ethical considerations

   Were the issues of informed consent, confidentiality, addressed? Was any harm or discomfort to individuals balanced against any benefits? Did an ethics committee approve the study?

7. Sample

   Who or what makes up the sample? Are there clear inclusion and exclusion criteria? What method of sampling was used? Are those in the sample typical and representative of the larger group, or are there any obvious elements of bias? On how many people/things/events are the results based?

8. Data presentation

   In what form are the results presented: tables, bar graphs, pie charts, raw figures, or percentages? Does the author explain and comment on these? Has the author used correlation to establish whether certain variables are associated with each other? Have tests of significance been used to establish to what extent any differences between groups/variables could have happened by chance? Can you make sense of the way the results have been presented, or could the author have provided more explanation?

(Continued)

> **BOX 5.1 Framework for critiquing quantitative research—cont'd**
>
> 9. Main findings
>   Which are the most important results that relate to the aim? (Think of this as putting the results in priority order; which is the most important result followed by the next most important result, etc. There may only be a small number of these.)
> 10. Conclusion and recommendations
>   Using the author's own words, what is the answer to the aim? If relevant, is the hypothesis accepted or rejected? Are the conclusions based on, and supported by, the results? What recommendations are made for practice? Are these relevant, specific and feasible?
> 11. Readability
>   How readable is it? Is it written in a clear, interesting style, or is it heavy going? Does it assume a lot of technical knowledge about the subject and/or research procedures (i.e. is there much unexplained jargon)?
> 12. Practice implications
>   Once you have read it, what is the answer to the question, 'so what'? Was it worth doing and publishing? How could it be related to practice? Who might find it relevant and in what way? What questions does it raise for practice and further study?

These might be found in the title, and most certainly in the aim. Ask yourself what is the basic theme of this article? The answer might be 'making informed choices', 'care of the perineum', or 'breastfeeding support'. Notice that these are not questions, nor are they long or detailed. We are looking at the broad canvas of which this study forms a part.

BACKGROUND

The opening to an article should provide a convincing justification for choosing the topic area. Here we should expect a clear argument or evidence as to why the topic is a problem, the nature and implications of that problem, and how it has been examined in the literature. A study should start with the identification of a problem.

The author may use the subheading *'Review of the literature'* (or *'Literature review'*) in which previous studies are examined. Some articles may contain only a summary or synopsis of previous work. Where possible, however, an author should provide a critical review of the literature. This should draw attention to both strengths and weaknesses of individual studies, and the literature overall. In this section the author may explicitly or implicitly draw together the theoretical or conceptual framework of the study. This will answer the question, 'which concepts or variables are seen as linked for the purpose of this study'. The review of the literature section should open with some indication of how the search for appropriate literature was conducted, for example the databases, key words and time frame used (see Chapter 6). These will help identify if a comprehensive review was conducted.

AIM (TERMS OF REFERENCE)

The background should prepare the way for the aim or 'terms of reference', which is the question the data will be collected to answer. There are two places where the aim can usually be found. The first is in the abstract, sometimes found underneath the title. The second place is just before the subheading, 'method'. Although the aim usually begin with the word 'to', sometimes because of the grammatical construction of the sentence we might have to insert it ourselves (e.g. if it says 'this study examines the problem, etc. we would insert 'to examine' the problem, etc.'). If the work is experimental there might also be a *hypothesis* or assumption the researcher is testing. The author's stated aim and hypothesis will help us identify if these were achieved or answered.

With the aim, and the hypothesis if present, it should be possible to identify which of the three levels of research question has been used (see Chapter 2). The study variable(s) should also be clear at this stage. Where the research question is level three, there will be dependent and independent variables, and the researchers should provide a concept and operational definitions for the variables. (It may be helpful to return briefly to Chapter 2 for a reminder of these terms and their meaning.)

In writing or producing a critique, it helps to use the author's own words, rather than paraphrase them, to avoid change their meaning. Try to both describe what you have found under each heading in the critique framework, and also say how well you feel the author has accomplished each aspect. In other words, it is not simply what they said but how well they said it. This will result in a critical analysis of the article.

METHODOLOGY

This section indentifies the research design of the project, and matches its suitability to the research question. The first stage is to classify it under one of the following:

- experimental design with an experiment and control group,
- correlation, where the researcher searchers for patterns or associations between variables,
- a survey where the purpose is description,
- a qualitative design where the purpose is to gain insights into people's perceptions, beliefs, or behaviour.

Do you feel there is a match between the design and the aim? Within the broad research approach, you will identify which tool of data collection has been used. What are some of the strengths and weakness of the tool of data collection that makes it appropriately chosen here? Are the limitations of that tool recognised? Has triangulation been used, where the author has used more than one method of data collection to look at the same variable? Has the researcher attempted to strengthen the accuracy or 'reliability' of the tool? For instance, has the researcher used a pilot study to check the consistency of the tool of data collection?

The critique will consider the ethical issues related to the tool of data collection. Here, we consider the principles of research governance (see Chapter 8), such as informed consent, confidentiality, and an evaluation of the possible negative consequences of taking part in the study. Has the researcher gained approval from an ethics committee or is it not appropriate in this case? In an increasing number of research publications, there may only be a comment that ethical approval has been given by an appropriate ethics committee. As these committees are very careful in giving permission to carry out a study, it can be assumed that all the other elements were therefore present, otherwise permission would not have been granted.

We should also examine the sample of people, events or objects involved in the study. Are there clear inclusion and exclusion criteria that will help us to consider if they were appropriate for the study (see Chapter 14)? We should also identify the total numbers on whom the results are based. Here, we need to be careful, as large numbers could be initially involved or targeted but, through a poor response rate, individuals dropping out, or being eliminated from analysis for one reason or another, the final numbers could be quite small. Our main concern with the sample is whether we feel it is typical of the group it represents. It is not only sample size but also geographical variations and characteristics of the sample that need consideration. Could there be cultural patterns related to the country or part of the country, or social class, that might also influence the results? What was the name of the method used to draw people into the study and does this have particular strengths or limitations? The wrong or inappropriate sampling strategy might seriously limit the extent to which findings may be generalised.

MAIN FINDINGS

In this section we are concerned with the result of the data collection. Main findings will have a reasonably large number attached to them, and which relate to the aim. Look at these in the light of what might be an anticipated response to questions or measurements against which we can compare the findings. For example, what proportion of women would we expect to have held the baby within 5 minutes of the birth? If we would expect in the region of 85%, and the results showed that only 48% of women held her baby within 5 minutes of the birth, we would consider this a main finding. In any study there may only be a small number of perhaps three or four main findings. How easy is it to pick these out?

The results section of studies can look intimidating, especially if we do not have a full understanding of some of the statistical terminology and symbols. However, it does not take long to learn some of these meanings, and the results section can become clearer once we have learnt a few of these (see Chapter 13). Although it is reasonable for authors to make some assumptions about the level of statistical knowledge readers of certain journals should possess, unfamiliar specialised terms and procedures should be clarified. If the author is interested in reaching the widest audience, these terms should be explained. The author should also highlight what is noteworthy from the tables and graphs, so the reader can understand the researcher's viewpoint. Understanding the results section can take time and perseverance but a critique cannot be made unless you are clear on the results of a study.

IN THE END

Following the results section, the author will present the issues that have arisen from the findings in the discussion. This section may also include the author's own comments on any limitations to the study, such as the size and composition of the sample, or the limitations of the tool of data collection. These comments should be seen as positive, and a demonstration of rigour, as the researcher is seeking to help the reader form a balanced view of the results. The discussion section will take some of the issues or implications raised by the results and present the author's interpretation of their relevance for the aim of the study. The discussion may also refer to the findings of other studies to compare or contrast with the findings in the study under review. While reading the discussion it is important to consider your own view of the arguments put forward. Do you agree, or are there other possible interpretations?

The discussion should be followed by the conclusion and provide an answer to the study's aim using or 'echoing' some of the same words as those used in the aim. Be on your guard for a 'conclusion' section that contains only recommendations. If this happens the 'real' conclusion may be hidden at the start of the discussion. Where the aim is made up of more than one part, question or hypothesis, each should have a clear conclusion. In our assessment, we must consider whether the conclusion was based on and supported by the results. Given the findings of the study, would we have come to the same conclusion? Is the evidence strong enough to support the conclusion, or are there alternative conclusions that the author has not considered?

The final element should be the recommendations. Sometimes these can be placed in a box or labelled as 'implications for practice'. What does the author suggest could improve the situation? Do these suggestions flow naturally from the discussion? Are the recommendations realistic and concrete or are they so vague and general that it is unlikely that improvements could be made? Do they give a clear idea of what the reader could go away and do, having read the report?

If we are to produce a critique of an article, there are two remaining categories we need to consider. The first is how would we describe its readability? Although research convention dictates the structure of a research article, report or presentation, this does not mean that it has to be dull and hard going to read or listen to. Although we may be more interested in a study that relates to our particular area of work or own interests, any study has the potential to be presented in an interesting way.

We should expect that a research article is written in a clear style, with a minimum of jargon. Complex terminology should be explained or clarified. However, the researcher should expect readers to be familiar with common research terms and to be prepared to look up unfamiliar terms known to the majority of readers.

Finally, the most important consideration is the application of the research to clinical practice. Once we have read the study, what is the answer to the question, 'so what'? What is the message for practice? Is there something that should happen now as a result of these findings? Perhaps we need to consider some of the points in the recommendations to see if there are some things that relate to our own activities or clinical area.

Once you applied all the sections in Box 5.1 to an article, you should feel that you have a clear understanding of how the author carried out the study. You should also feel that you have not accepted the author's work uncritically. Critiquing a research article is a meeting of minds: the researcher's and yours. The result should be a greater understanding and consideration of the topic under study.

Critiquing a research article should not automatically result in change. It may take a synthesis of other similar studies in the form of a literature review to produce sufficient evidence to change practice. A single study, however, could make us question what we do, and its effectiveness. We might start to think whether some of our knowledge has passed its 'sell-by-date' and whether we need to look at our practices more critically.

If we have conducted the critique fairly, we should be able to evaluate research from an informed and objective standpoint, and not reject it simply because it does not agree with our personal views. Midwives need to exercise the skill of critiquing for the benefit of all concerned. However, like all skills, it does need practice. As you work through this book, you will gain more and more knowledge to apply when critiquing. It is really helpful if you can discuss your critiques with others, perhaps in the form of a journal club. You should find that once you have used the framework for some time, you will begin to use the headings in your mind almost automatically, and you will not need to draw on the printed structure. You will then have reached the point where you have become an analytical consumer of research.

CRITIQUING QUALITATIVE RESEARCH

The aim of qualitative research, like that of quantitative research, is to increase our knowledge, and so improve practice. As a number of areas important to midwifery do not lend themselves to numeric results and statistical accuracy, other methodological approaches are applicable. Qualitative research is one such alternative (Chapter 4). It also allows us to identify those areas that women themselves value in relation to the care given to them by health professionals. This is an important element in improving the quality of care and the application of qualitative research as a source of evidence to improve care is already taking place in some areas of nursing (Hopkins 2010).

The last chapter emphasised that the differences in the way qualitative research is conducted and presented means that the use of a quantitative critiquing framework is not just difficult but in many ways inappropriate. Any attempt to use the quantitative approach to critiquing would inevitably lead to unfair criticism, as the way qualitative research is conducted appears to break many of the principles of quantitative research. These includes such things as a tool of data collection that is standardised and measures consistently, a variable that is open to quantification, the use of a pilot study to check the measuring accuracy of the data collection tool, or the use of a previous measuring tool, and a relatively large sample sizes – all of these are not found in qualitative research.

We need to adapt the critiquing framework to take account of these different principles and philosophy of research. This can be a challenge. Burns and Grove (2009), for instance, suggest that the first step is that the reader must be open and willing to move from often in-built assumptions of the quantitative world or paradigm of research to that of the qualitative researcher. They warn that this can involve setting aside personal and sometimes strongly held views as well thinking on a more conceptual basis to follow the inductive thinking of the qualitative researcher as they interpret the accounts gathered from participants. It is also clear that a qualitative critiquing framework should include some of the unique features of the research processes involved that differ considerably from those of quantitative research (McCarthy and O'Sullivan 2008). In this section some of these essential features are outlined and applied to a framework for critiquing qualitative studies (Box 5.2).

> **BOX 5.2 Framework for critiquing qualitative research**
>
> You should not expect to get answers to every question in each section, as what is important will vary from study to study. The questions provided here are to give you some guidance. (It is suggested that you photocopy this box, and use alongside relevant articles.)
>
> 1. Focus
>   What is the key issue, concept or problem the work examines? What are the key words you would file this article under? Are there clues to the focus in title? How important is this for practice and the profession? Is the type of qualitative design included in the title?
> 2. Background
>   What argument or evidence does the researcher provide for exploring this issue, concept or problem? Is there a review of previous literature on the subject or reference to government or professional reports that illustrate its importance? Are gaps in the literature or inadequacies with previous methods highlighted? Does the literature review examine the concepts or issues that form the focus? Is there an attempt to justify the study within the context of a qualitative research design? If this is grounded theory, there may not be a comprehensive review of the literature at this point, although some reference to previous work may be included as an illustration of its importance. There should be some argument or background information to justify looking at this particular subject.
> 3. Aim
>   What is the stated aim of the research? This will usually start with the word 'to'. There will not be a hypothesis or the identification of dependent and independent variables, as qualitative research answers a level-one question. There may be an attempt to provide a concept definition for the concept that forms the focus of the study. On the whole, you will find the aim very broad and general and not as detailed as in quantitative research.
> 4. Study design
>   There may be an acknowledgement that the study is qualitative in design and then the type of method specified. The main alternatives are 1. *phenomenological*, which explores what it is like to have a certain experience such as a birth, a pregnancy or threatened miscarriage, and how people interpret that experience; 2. *ethnographic*, where the researcher enters and participates in the world of the subject by listening, observing and asking questions in order to understand their view of the world; or 3. *grounded theory*, which will identify concepts which arise from the analysis of the data collected, and may also suggest a theory or hypothesis that explains or predicts some of the behaviour that has emerged in the study. It is important that the philosophy behind the method suits the intentions of the research.

(Continued)

BOX 5.2 Framework for critiquing qualitative research—cont'd

5. Tool of data collection

   Here we are interested not only in the technique used to collect the information, but the amount of detail we have on the circumstances under which the data were collected. This contributes to the credibility of the study. This should include details of the environment in which the data were collected, over what period of time data collection took place, and any other details that allow us to visualise the conduct of data collection. Did the researcher spend sufficient time, either in observing the life and behaviour of the subjects, or in interviewing subjects, to produce sufficient depth to the data? Because of the flexible way that data are gathered, and the way the method will change during data collection, a pilot study will not usually be employed. The researcher should, however, include detail of how they have attempted to achieve procedural rigour in the way the study was conducted. Did the researcher check with those in the study that the information collected was accurate (member's check)?

6. Ethical considerations

   As with qualitative studies, it is important that the researcher has protected the participant from harm, and has gained informed consent from those taking part in the study. It should not be possible to identify individuals or places where the study took place where this might affect anonymity. The researcher should illustrate ethical rigour, including, where appropriate, approaching a Local Research Ethics Committee (LREC), or in American studies an Institutional Review Board (IRB), to approve the research.

7. Sample

   Who forms the sample and what are their basic characteristics? The sample size may be quite small, even down to 3 or 4, but more usually about 10 to 15. This may be dictated by theoretical saturation, that is, data collection stops once no new themes or categories emerge from the analysis. In qualitative research, it is important to assess whether the participants possess the relevant knowledge or carry out the activity in which the researcher is interested. Has the researcher demonstrated that the participants are able to provide relevant information and are not open to any kind of bias? The reader must consider to what extent the findings, theory or conceptual categories may apply to other settings. This contributes to its *fittingness* to be applied elsewhere.

8. Data presentation

   The data will be presented in the form of description, dialogue or comments from participants. Is this 'thick' and 'rich' description? Is there sufficient detail for us to almost feel that we are there? Do the quotes from participants clearly illustrate the concepts they are being used to illustrate? Is there overdependence on comments from a small number of the participants in the sample? Have the researchers detailed how they ensured that the data were accurately recorded and representative of the data gathered? Is there anything about the circumstances in which the data were collected that could have threatened the accuracy of the data? Is it possible to discover the *'decision trail'* used by the researcher to determine how the raw data was processed into the categories presented in the results section? This contributes to its *auditability*. Given the same data, it should be possible, following the decision trail, to arrive at similar categories and conclusions. Does the researcher present the findings in the participant's own words rather than reinterpreting what was said or done?

BOX 5.2 Framework for critiquing qualitative research—cont'd

9. Main findings
   What are the key concepts or categories developed from the data? Do the concepts and categories presented cover all the data gathered? Were the findings checked either by the participants (member's check) or examined by other experts in the field (*peer review*)? Are the main findings credible, that is, have attempts been made to support the accuracy of the results through rigour in the way in which the study was conducted? Does the researcher discuss the findings and relate these to the literature, or do they leave the quotes to speak for themselves?
10. Conclusion
    Is there a clear answer to the aim? Does the researcher propose a relationship between the concepts and categories developed in the analysis to form a clear conceptual or theoretical framework? Does the conceptual or theoretical framework reflect the data? Has the conclusion been arrived at inductively (built up from the findings)?
11. Readability
    Does the researcher present the description of the social circumstances described in the research in sufficient detail that one can almost imagine being there, and hear the participants talking and carrying out the activities described? Is it possible to recognise the concepts described as related to practical experience? Is the report written in a simple and understandable way? Is there a clear 'story line' emerging from the research?
12. Relevance to practice
    Are the findings relevant to practice or professional knowledge? Is it an important area related to current concerns and issues within the profession? Does the research satisfy the criteria of *transferability*, that is, can the findings in the form of the theory, concepts or categories developed through the study be applied to other situations, or are they only applicable to the place and the people where the study took place? Do you feel the research has sensitised you to issues or provided further insight? Has it confirmed views you might have already held?

FOCUS, BACKGROUND AND AIM

Qualitative research often centres on a key human or social concept, issue or theme. As with quantitative research, the researcher should provide a clear rationale as to why the study has been undertaken. This will consist of the identification of important professional issues, local problems, or key concepts relevant to the profession or clinical practice. These concepts should be clearly defined in the background to the study. In the case of some forms of qualitative research, such as grounded theory, the researcher may avoid reading too much literature in detail prior to data collection. This is in case it directs the research too much and influences what is seen as key structures in the study. Qualitative researchers should allow the issues to arise naturally by participants to highlight what is important for them. In other qualitative studies, particularly those that do not take a grounded theory approach, the researcher might present a critical review of the literature, in the same way as quantitative studies. The researcher will state an aim, but this may be deliberately broad to provide flexibility and avoid preconceived ideas. It may well simply say the intention is to examine the experience or perception of some concept or other, such as the experience of a home birth or having a baby with a cleft palate. The question will not be at level two or three as each of those require numerical measurements to answer them.

METHODOLOGY

In outlining the methodology, the researcher should be as rigorous as the quantitative researcher, and illustrate the steps taken to make the process of data collection as accurate as possible. As an attempt is made to avoid separating those taking part from the social contexts in which they function, there should be rich or 'thick' descriptions of the setting. Holloway and Wheeler (2010: 7) suggest that 'thick' description involves a detailed portrayal of the participants' experiences that go beyond a surface reporting of phenomena, and which uncover feelings and the meanings given to their actions. This should produce a richly visual picture of what is going on, and so detailed that we almost feel ourselves to be there.

As the researcher attempts to be as flexible as possible in collecting the data there will rarely be a pilot study aimed at testing the measuring accuracy of the data collection tool. However, some researchers will carry out a number of 'practice' interviews to experience the response to the interviews or observations. These different approaches to data gathering raise the question of what evaluative criteria can be used to assess the quality of these studies. Whereas quantitative research is evaluated using the concepts of reliability, validity, bias and rigour, the flexibility of qualitative designs has led to a great debate as to whether any evaluative criteria can meaningfully be applied when critiquing them (Polit and Beck 2008, Holloway and Wheeler 2010). However, some methods of assessing studies should be considered. Here, we will draw on the criteria developed some time ago by Guba and Lincoln and cited by many other authors (Polit and Beck 2008, Schmidt and Brown 2009). The first of these is the concept of *trustworthiness*. This is an overarching term that Schmidt and Brown (2009: 307) define as follows:

> Trustworthiness refers to the quality, the authenticity, and the truthfulness of findings in qualitative research. It relates to the degree of trust, or confidence, readers have in the results.

Trustworthiness is said to have been satisfied if the following criteria can be satisfied:

- *Credibility* This relates to whether the details of the study are believable and appear accurate. This can be helped by the amount of description researchers provide and whether they have checked their data and interpretations with any of the participants to ensure they are 'recognised' by those involved as true and accurate. This technique is called a *'member's check'*, where those in the study confirm the accuracy of the researcher's transcription or interpretation. Other techniques include *'negative case analysis'* where the researcher deliberately looks at the findings for examples that do not fit their developing ideas and may then refine their categories, and keeping a *'reflective journal'* that captures ideas and thoughts to ensure they contribute to the analysis and interpretation process.

- *Dependability/Auditablity* This illustrates the researcher's decision-making process and allows the reader to see how they developed the category headings and themes from the analysis of the interviews or observations. The researcher should give examples of what was categorised under the theme headings, and the reader should have confidence in the extensive data that the researcher used to develop this analysis.
- *Confirmability* This provides support for the researcher's ideas to show they are not preconceived ideas or subjective views but can be shown to be taken from the findings of the study.
- *Transferability* Although qualitative research cannot be generalised to other situations in the same way as quantitative research, there is still a desire that the insights or interpretations may be useful in other settings.

All of these terms are abstract and therefore can seem confusing at first. However, you will find that many qualitative studies refer directly to these terms in their methods section in an attempt to demonstrate the rigour of their study, and your understanding of their meaning will increase.

The sample size of qualitative research tends to be much smaller than quantitative research as data collection is a more extensive for each person. In other words, the emphasis is the depth rather than breadth of data collection. The aim is not to produce a sample that is statistically similar to the larger population; the intention is to include those in a position to talk in an informed way about the concept of concern to the study. In qualitative research the researcher is often dependent on *'informants'* who volunteer information, or agree to provide an insider's view of things. We should expect, however, that there is an attempt to acknowledge and limit bias as much as possible so that a range of experiences or interpretations are covered by the sample. Once the researcher feels that subjects are revealing no new insights or themes, data collection may be ended on the grounds that *'data saturation'* has been reached, and further participants would not add anything new to the study.

The issue of ethics should also be addressed, as they are equally as important as in quantitative research. Here, the researcher ensures that the individual is not put at any disadvantage as a result of being part of the study and should gain informed consent from participants. Where appropriate, the Local Research Ethics Committee (LREC) will also be approached to give approval for the study. American studies will refer to an Institutional Review Board (IRB), which serves the same purpose.

ANALYSIS

In qualitative research, data analysis works in harmony at the same time as data collection. At this point, the researcher inductively analyses the findings for what they might reveal about the focus of the study. If the researcher is to avoid the accusation of bias and researcher subjectivity, it should be clear how decisions have been made throughout the research so that the reader can understand the thinking employed, not only in conducting the research, but also in the analysis of the findings. This element of *dependability* should take the form of an *'audit trail'* for the reader to follow, showing how the raw data have systematically and consistently led to category headings that have been applied in the same way for the same elements.

The results section of qualitative research is usually referred to as the *'findings'*, and differs from that of quantitative research as it will take the form of direct quotations, either from a participant or from a dialogue involving both a participant and the researcher. It may also include descriptions of places or events. In some instances, these will be extracts from the researcher's *'fieldwork diary'* or notebook.

Along with the presentation of this form of data, the findings section may also draw on the literature to support the credibility of the findings and their interpretation.

CONCLUSION

The conclusion of the study may give both the answer to the aim and also put forward a possible explanation or interpretation of the findings that result in the statement of a theory or a conceptual framework that may be explored by subsequent research.

APPLICATION TO PRACTICE

The reader of qualitative research will want to apply the research to clinical and professional practice. As one of the aims of qualitative research is to sensitise the reader to the position and experiences of those in the study, the application to practice will include the extent to which new insights and awareness have been achieved through reading the study. Although it is often assumed that the findings of qualitative research are not generalisable, the concept of *fittingness* suggests that there may be wider issues and principles that are transferable to other settings, providing the analysis relates to similar situations. The rigour relating to the way in which the research has been conducted will also be brought into question at this point, as the accuracy of the findings must be considered, and the extent to which any theoretical or conceptual frameworks really do fit the situation described.

This outline of the framework for qualitative research indicates that this form of research is no less rigorous than quantitative research. In the same way, the critical reader approaches the published work is no less systematic than with any other study.

CONDUCTING RESEARCH

This chapter is relevant to those undertaking research in two ways. Firstly, the skill of critiquing is an essential part of reviewing the literature, and therefore the researcher should approach the literature in a critical and analytical way. The frameworks in this chapter can be used by the researcher when considering the work of others. Secondly, researchers should remember that when they publish the results of their study, it will be subjected to the type of scrutiny suggested here. If researchers are aware of the criteria and framework that readers will use to evaluate their work, then they can ensure that these areas are addressed when writing up their study.

In the section on qualitative research, it has been emphasised how important it is for researchers to paint a very clear and vivid picture of their experience in conducting the study. This process is facilitated through the use of a fieldwork diary, or field notes (Polit and Beck 2008). These should contain all the essential descriptive elements relating to the fieldwork. They should also contain the major analytical processes that unfolded throughout data analysis. It is from these that the researcher can clearly demonstrate the decision trail by illuminating how the different conceptual categories arose from the mass of findings.

CRITIQUING RESEARCH

This chapter has focused on the need to question and critically analyse published research. If practice is to be evidence-based, all practitioners must develop analytical skills to allow them to assess the quality of evidence available for decision making. This should not be a purely negative activity, but should take a balanced view, identifying both the strengths and weaknesses of the work. Remember, research is a difficult activity and it is important to identify the limitations of a study whilst recognising the constraints under which research is conducted.

It is important that the appropriate critiquing format has been used on the research. There is no use applying the quantitative critiquing framework on a qualitative article or vice versa. This chapter has attempted to provide suitable frameworks for each of these research approaches so you can critique articles, and research reports, and even verbal research presentations and posters. You might find it useful to photocopy the two tables so that you have a more readily accessible checklist to follow when critiquing.

KEY POINTS

- Research is rarely conducted under perfect conditions and so weaknesses can be found in most published research. This means that, just because a piece of research has been published, it is not above constructive criticism.
- Critiquing research articles should be accomplished using a systematic approach. This chapter has provided two critique frameworks: one for quantitative research articles, and the other for qualitative articles. As these two designs are based on different principles, it is important that the criteria for judging one form are not applied to the other.
- A critique should have a balance between description – what the researcher(s) did, and analysis – how well it was done. Undertaking a critique provides a sound basis for establishing evidence-based practice as it ensures that published research is carefully evaluated and not accepted on face value.

REFERENCES

Burns, N., Grove, S., 2009. The Practice of Nursing Research: Appraisal, Synthesis, and Generation of Evidence, sixth ed. Saunders, St Louis.

Holloway, I., Wheeler, S., 2010. Qualitative Research for Nurses, third ed. Wiley-Blackwell, Chichester.

Hopkins, A., 2010. Using qualitative research to improve tissue viability care. Nurs. Stand. 24 (32), 64–67.

Lavender, T., 2010. Is there enough evidence to meet the expectations of a changing midwifery agenda. In: Spiby, H., Munro, J. (Eds.), Evidence-Based Midwifery: Applications in Context. Wiley-Blackwell, Chichester.

McCarthy, G., O'Sullivan, D., 2008. Evaluating the literature. In: Watson, R., McKenna, H., Cowman, S., Keady, J. (Eds.), Nursing Research: Designs and Methods. Churchill Livingstone, Edinburgh.

Polit, D., Beck, C., 2008. Nursing Research: Generating and Assessing Evidence for Nursing Practice, eighth ed. Lippincott Williams and Wilkins, Philadelphia.

Schmidt, N., Brown, J., 2009. Evidence-Based Practice for Nurses: Appraisal and Application of Research. Jones and Bartlett, Sudbury.

Reviewing the literature

A review of the literature can be defined as the critical examination of a defined selection of published literature on a particular topic or issue. According to Murphy and Cowman (2008) its purpose is to produce a picture of what is currently known about a problem or situation and to identify what knowledge gaps may exist. A review of the literature is not simply a task carried out by researchers; it has now become an important part of evidenced-based practice as well as a familiar activity in many educational course assignments. The aim of this chapter is to provide practical advice on producing critical reviews of the literature suitable for many situations.

The process of reviewing the literature has changed considerably over time from a simple summary of what some of the literature says to a critical evaluation and synthesis of carefully sourced high-quality research evidence that can be used to support clinical decision making. However, we will start with the following simple definition:

A review of the literature is the systematic and critical examination of a defined selection of published literature on a particular topic or issue.

The key aspects highlighted in this definition are that reviews must be planned very carefully to provide the best-quality evidence, and that evidence should be subject to critical analysis to ensure that the findings are sound and transferable to practice. Reviews come in a number of forms, such as the following suggested by Mileham (2009):

- *Narrative*: where the emphasis is on summarising the literature,
- *Integrated*: where a critical evaluation of key studies are brought together in a systematic way,
- *Meta-analyses*: where similar types of quantitative studies are combined statistically to try to overcome the problem of small sample sizes,
- *Systematic review*: where a strict system of selecting and extracting key information is used by teams of reviewers to ensure only the highest quality to inform evidence-based practice.

© 2011 Elsevier Ltd. All rights reserved.

In addition to the meta-analysis of quantitative studies a similar process is carried out with qualitative studies referred to as meta-synthesis or meta-studies (Ploeg 2008). In evidence-based practice the most sophisticated and highly sought source of evidence is the systematic review. This is because of the strict quality control placed on the studies included and the expertise of those who conduct them. In most academic courses and clinical settings the goal is usually a well-conducted integrated review that critically evaluates the studies. Such reviews rarely cover the kind of material included in systematic reviews such as the *grey literature* (conference papers and theses). This chapter will mainly focus on the skills involved in the integrated review.

Why carry out a review? There are perhaps four main reasons for reviewing the literature, two of which are clinical and two academic:

- as part of clinical effectiveness where clinicians search for evidence of best practice on which to base clinical decisions,
- as the basis for standards, protocols and guidelines for practice that will later lead to an audit of 'best practice' based on the review,
- as part of the research process where its purpose is to inform the researcher on the present state of knowledge on the topic to be covered by the study and to locate the current study within the context of that knowledge,
- as an integral part of a student assignment, or as the main focus of an assignment or dissertation for an educational course.

This demonstrates that reviews are not simply, as Mileham (2009) points out, an academic exercise left behind at the end of a course; they are an essential skill for all health professionals.

The method of producing a review will be different within each of these four activities. In the educational setting, the depth of analysis will vary by the academic level of the course or programme of study. Most academic levels now encourage critical analysis and not just a summarising of content. At dissertation level, the depth of analysis will be paramount and the research knowledge of the student should be clearly demonstrated. The dissertation will also concentrate on a far greater conceptual or abstract level of analysis, often relating the literature to a theoretical or conceptual framework. In the clinical setting, the review will seek best practice for an activity or choice of intervention. In the research context, reviews are produced for a number of reasons, listed by Holloway and Wheeler (2010: 36) as:

- to find out what is already known about the subject and acknowledge those who have worked in this area,
- to identify gaps in the knowledge,
- to describe how the study contributes to existing knowledge of a topic area,
- to avoid duplicating other people's work,
- to assist in defining the research question,
- to place the research in the context of other studies,
- to show that the researcher has reflected on the research question.

THE PROCESS OF REVIEWING THE LITERATURE

Producing a rigorous review of the literature consists of the following three stages, each with its own demands and skills required to accomplish them:

- sourcing, or searching for and locating appropriate literature,
- evaluating the results of the search and extracting relevant detail,
- writing the review based on the synthesis and evaluation of the material.

There are surprising similarities between conducting a review of the literature and a research project; both start with a precise question, and maximum effort must go into the planning stage. A statement such as: *'I want to find out about women who have twins'* is unlikely to be successful. Try to be clear on the question you want the review to answer. A more suitable wording would be *'What are the main physical, psychological and social problems faced by women who have twins?'* Even this may be too ambitious for one assignment or review and just one of those three aspects may be more appropriate.

The review, when written, will consist of a number of subheadings under which you will group or 'cluster' the literature. The key words that may prompt you to clarify the headings under which the review will be structured are listed in Box 6.1.

Not all of these would be used for every subject. If we take the example of reviewing the literature on twins discussed above, we can see how they can be applied in practice. The process of planning the review may follow similar lines to that outlined in Box 6.2.

If at this stage it is evident that the review is going to be large, the scope can be reduced to look at an aspect of it, such as the consequence of birthing twins in the first 3 months following birth. In this way the planning stage helps to clarify the question that the review will answer. It is also important to realise that some of the above questions will vary in emphasis. This will have implications for the amount of space devoted to exploring them. The answers to some questions will be discussed in a sentence or two; others will be several pages long.

BOX 6.1 Key words that may help to identify suitable theme headings for structuring a review

What (definitions of key terms or concepts)
Why (what are the causes/influences of the key term/concept)
Who (is particularly affected/at risk/involved)
When (are there particular times when this might happen or action ought to be taken)
How (does it happen/take place/can we do something about it)
Problems
Solutions/recommendations
Advantages
Disadvantages
Implications for practice

> **BOX 6.2 Planning a review of the literature**
>
> Aim of the review:
>   To consider the physical, psychological and social implications of the birth of twins on the mother and family, and to identify the implications of these factors for the midwife.
> Possible theme headings:
> *What* are twins – how is this clinically defined, what variations are there?
> *Why* do twins occur – what are the factors associated with twin pregnancies?
> *Who* is most likely to have twins?
> *When* should some of the implications be considered?
> *How* do twins influence physical, psychological, social factors related to the mother and family?
> *Problems* – what problems are associated with twins in pregnancy, birth, and early months?
> *Solutions* – how can some of the identified problems he reduced?
> *What* are the *implications* for the midwife and maternity services?

The structure of the review may be reassessed as the material is gathered. For instance, it may be better to put some of the material such as the 'what is meant by…' in an introduction. The main body of the review may concentrate on the two headings of *'the main problems faced by the mothers of twins'* and *'ways in which problems can be reduced'*. A final heading may then be *'implications for practice'*. This would consider what the literature suggests are possible steps that need to be taken and would not be the writer's views. The review has to be located squarely in the literature and not take an 'essay' style coming mainly from the writer using some apt quotes to support the writer's arguments. As a suggestion, the main section of the review should be written under about three to five theme headings, but this is only a very general guideline.

SOURCING THE LITERATURE

Once we have a clear question to answer, we can set about finding or *'sourcing'* the literature. A review is only as good as the quality of the literature on which it is based, so this phase must be accomplished to a high standard. Mileham (2009) acknowledges that this aspect is time consuming, but knowing how to make effective use of databases and search engines can reduce the time and effort required. This section will explain some of the principles in gathering relevant references quickly and making judgements on what is worth using in the review.

Firstly, reviews draw, in the main, on journal articles. This is because journals are usually more up to date than books. The key principle is to use only the full text of articles as the basis for a review. You should not use the 'abstract' of an article, that is, the short summary written under the title and used in databases to provide a quick overview. Relying on the abstract is likely to be very misleading as it is an incomplete view of the article. How can you make a valid assessment of only an incomplete part of something?

In sourcing the literature, the first stage is to write a clear question you will answer through the review, and then break this down into the key words or variables that may help you search for relevant literature. It is useful once you have the key words to write below them alternative terms to describe the same situation (synonyms) so that you can use all the alternatives to maximise your search strategy. You should also list any possible variations in spelling, especially with American variations such as 'labor' (US) and 'labour' (UK). The trick is to think of this as finding the door behind which the information you need is kept, where each door has a variety of words used to describe its contents. Your task is to discover which words will open the maximum number of words for you. For example, 'teenage' as in 'teenage pregnancies', may have synonyms such as 'adolescent, 'young people', and '13–18 years'. Similarly, 'antenatal education' may have synonyms such as 'parentcraft', 'childbirth education' or 'parenting education'. Some of these options may be listed automatically by some databases under 'subject' headings where a range of words used to store this information is listed. Some databases will then allow you to build up your search by gradually adding the various search terms so that all the search terms are added together and the database will display articles for the combined words. This results in the number of hits being reduced as it excludes duplicate articles or articles that do not include the combination of words.

As there are a number of possible databases to search, decisions must be made on which ones may be more appropriate to search for a particular topic. Topics of a more clinical nature will be covered in databases such as 'The Cochrane Library' and 'MEDLINE', whereas more professional issues or woman-centred issues will be more likely in CINAHL or British Nursing Index (BNI). For midwifery issues, the MIDIRS website should also be included. Do not simply search one database, as each one is designed to cover a slightly different aspect, and no database is complete. You will be expected to demonstrate that you have undertaken a comprehensive search by searching across a number of databases.

In writing a review of the literature, it is customary to name the databases and the key words used to find the literature in a review, and any inclusion/exclusion criteria for articles (e.g. only UK articles, or excluding articles on babies in neonatal units), and the time frame used to search (how far back your search extends, e.g. 5 or 10 years). Some articles that have reviewed the literature also include the number of articles found ('hits') in various databases, and the numbers rejected for stated reasons. It is important, then, to think ahead and record these details so that, if required, you can clearly demonstrate how you arrived at the articles in your review. It will help to be systematic in your own records by building up a table for yourself where you can record the date of a search, the databases, search terms and the number of hits and references retrieved (Booth et al. 2010). As you build up your search of key words on a particular database, you may be able to save or print out the search details to allow you to record this information. The search details should include sufficient information for someone to follow reasonably closely in your footsteps.

It is worth being clear here on the distinction between databases and search engines. Search engines, which include such well-known names as 'Google' and 'Google Scholar' do not keep their own lists of articles but sweep the web to locate references and sometimes locate the original article for you to download or print, while a database is a listing of articles and their abstracts, and may or may not offer a link to download the article. In academic work, the emphasis is on databases such as CINAHL and British Nursing Index, as the journals they list tend to be those that have been *'peer reviewed'*, that is, they have been filtered first to ensure that they achieve a high quality. If practice is to be evidence-based it must be built on high-quality evidence articles, otherwise the wrong conclusion may be made. This is why your reviews should be based only on full *'primary references'*, that is, complete articles written by the authors of a study themselves; avoid the use of *'secondary references'*, that is, someone talking about or summarising another author's work, as you have thus not read the original and you are not in a position to personally judge its value.

One useful technique in searching for clues for relevant literature is *'back chaining'*. This involves finding one article relevant to your topic, either as a 'hard' paper copy or as a database search, and checking its list of references. The reference lists of these articles are then checked for further suitable articles, and so on. Once this has been completed several times you should find the same names keep appearing. These are the references you must try to locate, as they are the ones that play a major part in our understanding of the topic.

An alternative to 'back chaining' is *'forward chaining'*, where titles offered in databases offer the option, 'cited by' or 'similar references'. This means that a more recent author has mentioned the work of the author you are currently considering. Choosing this option will take you forward in time to a possibly relevant article.

At the end of this stage of searching the literature, the reviewer may be faced with one of two problems to overcome. The first is a shortage of useful articles, that is, when there are very few 'hits'. In these cases it is worth checking that relevant or accurate search terms have been used. The problem may just be a typing or spelling error. If the word appears to be correct, then it could be that the database keeps the information under a different key word. Try an alternative word. Asking library staff for suggestions is always useful, or if you have any articles on the subject, check if they list key words that the article has been listed under and try those. If this still does not produce many references, you may need to broaden the topic to include a wider subject of which your key word may form a part.

The second problem you may be faced with is the opposite of the above, where you have far too many hits, and are faced with 'information overload'. Here, you may have to limit the search in some way. One alternative is to reduce the time frame covered by the review to fewer years. You could also try to reduce the topic by taking one aspect of it rather than the whole topic. So if you are looking for information giving, you may limit it to the antenatal period rather than information giving in general.

Before we leave this section, it is important to recognise that databases can be challenging. The way they 'think' and operate can take some time to work out and so lead to feelings of frustration. Remember, using these resources is a skill, and it does take some practice. One solution is to get the help of colleague who is proficient or arrange with library staff for a personal demonstration.

EXTRACTING RELEVANT DETAILS

At the end of the sourcing phase, you should have a reasonable number of references on which to base your review. Once you physically have your articles, either as a paper copy or electronic copy, it is time to critically assess the material and extract relevant information for your review. To achieve this, you will need to examine all the articles systematically using a critiquing system such as the ones provided in Chapter 5. It is important to state that a review is not written as a series of critiques placed back to back. You need to compare and contrast different studies and comment on the importance of these for the question that forms the aim of the review in the process of synthesis. You do not have to wait for all the articles to be collected before starting this stage. You should start evaluating the studies as you get hold of them, as this may lead you in different and productive directions.

Given the possibly large number of articles forming the basis of the review, we can understand the point made by Polit and Beck (2008) that literature reviews are very complex and therefore extracting information should be carried out using a systematic process. During the initial stage of going through each article, one popular system is to use a fluorescent highlighter pen to mark key passages in paper copies of articles. Although this is useful as a preliminary stage, it is not helpful at the writing stage. This is because highlighter pens can be overused and you can be left with very few lines on a page that do not have a bright yellow (or alternative colour) line through it! As a result, important points can be difficult if not impossible to relocate.

How can we improve on the use of highlighted text? One answer is transfer the relevant text to a word file of quotes. You can put these under different theme headings in the word file. Always ensure you have recorded the author and page number if you combine quotes from different authors. It is useful to add your own comment underneath each one, saying what you feel about the comment or how you might use it in the review. This will allow you build up your analysis of the literature and already be developing a critical and analytical approach.

An alternative is to use a table or grid similar to a spreadsheet and use the columns to store useful quotes or information. If you examine some review of the literature articles, you will find that they use something similar in either the body or appendix. Each column in the table or grid (you will find 'landscape' a better format than 'portrait') should contain a theme or category heading that will be useful for comparisons. Although these headings may vary depending on the themes or issues in your review, where articles are research, you will find the headings used in Figure 6.1 will provide you with some useful ideas.

When reading an article or report it is possible to skim, or speed-read, until material relevant to one of the headings in the table is encountered. The material is then read slowly and a decision made as to whether any, or some, of the passage should be entered in the grid. When writing the review, details and comparisons between studies can be easily seen and used as the basis for critical analysis and comment. Sections or the entire table may be used in the body of the review, or included in an appendix.

Author (year)	Aim	Design & data collection tool	Sample number and selection method	Results	Conclusions	Recommendations	Your comments on strengths limitations
Author 1							
Author 2							
Etc.							

FIG 6.1 Literature extraction sheet for use with research studies

COMMON QUESTIONS

One of the most frequent questions asked by students writing a review is *'how many articles do I need for my review'*. Unfortunately, there is no magic number. The advice is to obtain as many articles as you can in as short a period of time as possible. The more articles you gather, the easier it will be to see a pattern under the various columns in your summary table. If time is limited, there should be two main priorities: include as much recent material as possible, as these will contain current thinking and evidence, and secondly, include as many of the 'classics' as possible. The latter are the titles that appear in the majority of writers' work on a particular topic.

A second question is *'how far back do I need to go'*. The usual guide is to go back approximately 5 years. If there is a lot of material, that may be sufficient, but if there is very little material, go back further. However, it is unwise to go further than 10 years for material other than classic or seminal work, as changes in health care and social factors mean that information will have passed its 'sell-by date' and be difficult to apply to the present.

A further question is *'do all the articles have to be research articles'*. The answer to this is that it is acceptable to include some descriptive reports based on individual thoughts, opinions or experiences, as well as policy documents, but, where possible, concentrate on research articles as they are the result of a more systematic process. The review question is important in guiding you to the kind of articles that will provide answers for the question.

A final question is *'can I use reviews of the literature in my own review'*. The answer is 'yes', as they provide high-quality evidence, but they will need to be carefully evaluated for their quality, as with all other articles. Previous reviews may differ in the question they asked compared to yours or have included more or different outcome measures to the ones in which you are interested. There is also the issue of age, as other articles, which you will include, may have emerged since the reviews.

WRITING THE REVIEW

Writing a critical review of the literature is a high-level skill. It is not simply a collection of quotes 'cut out' of the literature and pasted together, nor is it a series of critiques of individual research articles. It should contain both description of the content of studies and analysis and reflection on what they contain, how well it is presented, and how it all relates to the question the review will answer. The real essence of a good review of the literature is illustrated in the following comment from Burns and Grove (2009: 92):

> *The purpose is not to list all the material published, but rather to synthesize and evaluate it based on the focus of the review.*

In other words, the published work is not just presented in turn but woven together to show what different authors say or have found on the same aspects, and includes your views of the strengths of the studies based on your understanding of research processes and issues. It is this approach to reviewing the literature that gains the marks in written assignments based on literature reviews.

In terms of style, it should present a balanced view, looking at those studies that might support opposing views and look at the strength of evidence or argument presented. They should be written to demonstrate that you have been fair in presenting the evidence and have not let personal biases influence how the studies are presented. The review should be written under theme headings and provide readers with the body of the evidence that has been examined and help them understand the relative importance of the key papers and any limitations. In this way you should demonstrate ownership of the knowledge presented. It is not a summary of all the studies, but a careful analytical presentation of the studies you have presented. All the time you should be using the approach of:

DESCRIBE → COMPARE → CONTRAST → COMMENT

In this way there should be a balance between description and critical evaluation. The question driving the review should be foremost throughout, so that the reader does not have to keep thinking, 'How does this study fit in?' The relevance of studies should be made clear, and their contribution to the evidence judged in the light of other studies or views.

One important caution is to avoid being overconfident on the results of studies. Since the perfect conditions in which to conduct research rarely exist, there is rarely a situation where you would say this study 'proves'. Rather you would say, the study 'presents strong evidence', or 'supports the view that' something is the case. It is worth looking closely at reviews of the literature for the range of phrases and ways of writing the review so that you build up a repertoire of useful phrases and well chosen words.

At this stage, it is possible to suggest a systematic process to follow that takes into consideration all three sections covered so far. This is presented in Box 6.3.

CONDUCTING RESEARCH

A thorough review of the literature increases the researcher's ability to plan research effectively and efficiently. So much can be learned from the published work of others, both in terms of content (what has already been established) and process (how others have gone about exploring this topic). Research must be set within the context of current studies, so it is important that the review is comprehensive. The researcher should ensure that the review is based on a clear and well thought out search strategy. There should be an emphasis on more recent research, as this will provide information on the latest findings, understandings and approaches. Classic or seminal work should also be included.

The researcher should consider the literature critically, and compare and contrast the views and findings of key authors. This should be considered in relation to the aim of the intended research. In particular, examine concepts with their operational definitions, and the experiences of using data collection tools. The method of data analysis and presentation should also be considered for the way in which they might guide your study.

The review of the literature plays a key role in developing the tool of data collection. The main elements or variables identified as important in the literature will be reflected in the tool of data collection. Similarly, the literature review will guide the development of a theoretical or conceptual framework for the study.

BOX 6.3 The process of reviewing the literature

1. Decide on a clear question you want to answer through the review.
2. Plan the structure of the review by thinking of the themes that will be applicable. Remember that the following are useful starting points: what, why, when, who, how, problems and solutions or advantages and disadvantages, implications for practice.
3. Decide on the key words you may need for the topic along with synonyms and alternative spellings.
4. Identify a search strategy by listing possible sources references. Explore key databases such as CINAHL, MIDIRS, or The Cochrane Library. Be creative and use backward and forward chaining; use colleagues, other students, people in education, and specialists in the topic.
5. If there seems too little material, broaden the topic; if there is too much, focus the topic down to one aspect.
6. Decide on a time period (frame) to be covered; initially this could be 5 years. If there is too little, go back further; where there is too much reduce the number of years. Remember, it might be wise to include the classic (seminal) work.
7. As you locate material, whether it is articles, books or reports, ensure that all the information for a complete reference is recorded, or use a referencing computer programme.
8. Read through the material with your theme headings in mind. Scan fast until you meet with relevant material and then slow down and decide whether to extract it.
9. Enter the important material onto a grid or summary table. Don't forget your own comments on the material.
10. Examine your material for patterns by comparing and contrasting different authors.
11. Write a rough draft under the theme headings. Make sure you have both description (what the various authors say) as well as analysis (how well they say it). Make connections between the material for your reader, and relate studies and points to the purpose of the review. Keep telling the reader why the material included is relevant so they are not left thinking 'so what'.
12. When you are ready for the main draft, write a clear introduction including the question you set out to answer through the literature and describe your search strategy, which includes the databases, key words, time frame, the parameters used to select the material (the source of the material, e.g. British or British and American), and the themes used to group the literature.
13. At the end, make sure you relate the conclusion to practice. What can we say now, based on the literature? The conclusion should comment not only on the subject and what has been learnt, but also on the literature as a body of work itself. Is the available literature comprehensive, or are there gaps? Is the research of a high standard and rigorous, or does it contain weaknesses?
14. Remember, a review is not an essay that puts forward your views supported selectively by the literature. Neither is it a series of critiques. In writing the review, you should always start from the literature. What does it say?

Although, in the case of qualitative research, there is a feeling that reviewing the literature early on could 'contaminate' the research process, Holloway and Wheeler (2010) believe it is dangerous to start any study without some exploration of the literature on a topic, and support its use in the early stages of developing a research proposal, providing that it does not direct the research in too great a detail. In conducting research, then, the literature review is a fundamental building block of the research process, particularly in quantitative research.

CRITIQUING RESEARCH

When critiquing a research article, the review of the literature section can provide vital information on what stimulated the researcher's thinking. The design and the nature of the research question will have been influenced by what the researchers discovered in their review. This should be clearly evident in the article.

Some of the preliminary pointers the reader should consider include the extent of the review – how much literature is included and how up to date it is. Is there any area obviously missing? In particular, the reader should consider the extent to which the writers critically review the available literature. Do they identify strengths, weaknesses, and particularly gaps in the literature that will be addressed in their study?

The review of the literature should inform the reader and provide a clear rationale for conducting the study. Reading the review should provide an understanding of some of the key issues related to the topic and should also indicate some of the research that has already been undertaken in the area. In some cases, the review will also support the theoretical or conceptual framework that has been used in a study. This will link the key concepts together to show how they relate to each other.

KEY POINTS

- A review of the literature is the critical analysis of good-quality relevant work on a topic.
- Carrying out a review has a great deal to offer individual midwives and clinical areas in increasing the standard of evidence-based practice; it is also the focus of many student assignments and theses.
- Reviewing the literature is a skill that can be developed by following the principles outlined in this chapter.
- Sourcing the literature is influenced firstly by the identification of the relevant key words that allow access to the literature through databases. A search strategy should be produced at the start of the search and a record kept of the experiences with the databases.
- It is important to be systematic in the method of retrieving information from individual books and articles.
- In writing the review, the topic should be presented under relevant themes.
- A review of the literature is not a series of critiques joined together but an examination of the body of knowledge on a stated topic following the selection criteria stated in the review.
- If a review is to be relevant to practice, it should include both description and critical analysis. It should end with clear recommendations for practice.

REFERENCES

Booth, A., Rees, A., Beecroft, C., 2010. Systematic reviews and evidence syntheses. In: Gerrish, K., Lacey, A. (Eds.), The Research Process in Nursing, sixth ed. Wiley-Blackwell, Chichester.

Burns, N., Grove, S., 2009. The Practice of Nursing Research: Appraisal, Synthesis, and Generation of Evidence, sixth ed. Saunders, St Louis.

Holloway, I., Wheeler, S., 2010. Qualitative Research for Nurses, third ed. Wiley-Blackwell, Chichester.

Mileham, P., 2009. Finding sources of evidence. In: Schmidt, N., Brown, J. (Eds.), Evidence-Based Practice for Nurses: Appraisal and Application of Research. Jones and Bartlett, Sudbury.

Murphy, P., Cowman, S., 2008. Accessing the nursing research literature. In: Watson, R., McKenna, H., Cowman, S., Keady, J. (Eds.), Nursing Research: Designs and Methods. Edinburgh, Churchill Livingstone.

Ploeg, J., 2008. Identifying the best research design to fit the question Part 2: qualitative research. In: Cullum, N., Ciliska, D., Haynes, R., Marks, S. (Eds.), Evidenced-Based Nursing: An Introduction. Blackwell, Oxford.

Polit, D., Beck, C., 2008. Nursing Research: Generating and Assessing Evidence for Nursing Practice, eighth ed. Lippincott Williams and Wilkins, Philadelphia.

The research question

Midwifery has no shortage of questions that need to be answered. However, constructing a sound and researchable question is an art that takes practice, and the observation of a number of principles. Careful thought is essential, as the success of a project is measured against the question it set out to answer. The research question, then, is the gateway into the heart of the research process; the researcher must get this stage right, as so many other parts of the research process are influenced by it.

But where do research questions come from and what makes a good question? This chapter will outline their importance, and address some of the issues relating to their construction. The purpose of a hypothesis will also be examined, and the different forms they take will be outlined.

THE ROLE OF THE RESEARCH QUESTION

If we compare research to setting out on a journey, then the research question is the statement of the destination. We cannot map a clear and effective route unless we know where we are going, and we certainly will not know whether we have arrived, unless we know where we wanted to be at the end of the journey. In the same way, the research question allows the researcher to plan the research in the best possible way, and make important decisions to ensure that the correct destination is reached.

The following are aspects of the research process that will be influenced by the research question:

- the broad research approach (design),
- the tool of data collection (the method),
- the sample,
- the form of data analysis,
- the ethical considerations.

We can see now what Atkinson (2008: 67) had in mind when he said:

> *Developing a clear research question is the key to the development of any research investigation...*

© 2011 Elsevier Ltd. All rights reserved.

Research questions evolve from the choice of a particular topic area. This is often a topic felt to be problematic or where questions are raised on what is best practice for optimum care. The choice of topic can emerge from a desire to improve the quality of services, whilst others arise from reviewing the literature, or from searching for ways to provide clinically effective care. In fact, according to Houser (2008), the search for research problems is one of the easiest parts of the research process, and that is certainly true within midwifery.

Can research answer every kind of question? The answer is 'no'. Some questions demand a value judgement for their resolution, and are not open to research. For example, 'Should midwives carry out some of the more technological procedures currently performed by obstetricians?' Although we can survey midwives' views or those of obstetricians, the answers would not indicate whether it is 'right', only what people feel about it. Similarly, some questions are ethical or philosophical questions and cannot be answered by research but need to be discussed and debated.

Further light is shed on this issue by Burns and Grove (2009: 76) who propose that questions about practice fall into three categories:

- questions answered by existing knowledge,
- questions answered with problem solving,
- research-generating questions.

The first option is important as it illustrates that we should not rush into research without checking whether there is already knowledge available to answer our question. That is why a review of the literature is such an important preliminary stage to starting research. Their second category relates to the need for debate, reflection and problem solving. The third category is the one in which we are interested.

One important consideration before pursuing a research question is that of relevance. Does the research need to be done? Every research idea should be evaluated in terms of the contribution it will make to midwifery: 'Do we need to know the answer to the question?' This can be characterised as the 'so what' and 'who cares' test, which ensures that thought it given to the outcome of research and its relevance to practice, the development of theory or its contribution to shaping policy.

Perhaps the most important criteria in judging the relevance of a research project is whether women, their babies and their family gain from this research? Even if the topic relates to midwives themselves, those receiving care may still benefit indirectly through an increase or change in midwives' knowledge, skills or attitudes.

Having considered the relevance of a particular study, the next issue is that of feasibility. This includes such factors as:

- availability of time,
- availability of funding and resources,
- ethical consideration,
- researcher expertise,
- participant availability and willingness to take part,
- cooperation of key decision makers such as clinicians and managers who will be affected by the data-gathering process and its possible disruptive effect and economic cost.

The researcher must be able to confirm that all of these issues can be successfully addressed before the research can go any further.

TYPES OF RESEARCH QUESTIONS

Research questions are structured in a number of different ways according to the level of question (Wood and Ross-Kerr 2006) (see Chapter 2). The way the question is written or 'framed' will illustrate the level it addresses. Each level is associated with an appropriate broad research approach. For example, a level-one question will suggest the use of a survey or a qualitative approach such as an ethnographic or phenomenological study. Level-one questions are those where little is known about a topic and the intention is to describe a situation. There is only one variable in a level-one question. The researcher should give a clear concept definition that relates to the way the variable will be defined for the purposes of the study. There should also be an operational definition in a quantitative study that will outline the way it is intended to measure that variable. At this level there is no attempt to establish cause-and-effect relationships between variables.

A level-two question may also suggest a survey, but the question will be concerned with the pattern or correlation between variables. This level may also involve the collection of physiological measurements through observation or taking samples where at least two different measures from each subject are compared statistically to see if they show a similar pattern or correlation. In a level-two question more is known about the topic. Here, the purpose of the research is to establish if there is a statistical relationship in the form of a correlation between the variables that have been identified. At this level, according to Wood and Ross-Kerr (2006), although the researcher might have a shrewd idea of what to expect, there is not enough firm evidence from a randomised control trial to confidently predict an outcome and so achieve a level-three question.

A level-three question will look for a cause-and-effect relationship between two variables, particularly in relation to a clinical outcome. In a level-three question there will be enough known about the nature of the relationship between the variables in the study to make a confident prediction about relationships and outcomes. The purpose is to examine why a relationship exists, or to test a theory. This is achieved by manipulating the independent variable to measure its effect on the dependent variable in an experimental design study such as a randomised control trial. Some of the questions midwifery research attempts to answer and how these are related to the level of question are shown in Table 7.1.

Examining the research questions will also suggest a particular method of data collection that might accurately answer the question. Although in many cases a choice may exist, such as the use of questionnaires or interviews, the nature of some questions will suggest which method might be more appropriate. So, if the question is broad or more abstract, or if it is a delicate or sensitive topic, an exploratory interview will be more appropriate than a questionnaire. Conversely, if the question requires specific and basic information, particularly where the likely responses fall into a small number of choices, a questionnaire will be a more appropriate method of collecting the data on the grounds of speed, cost and ease of analysis. If the question is about behaviour, then, providing it is feasible and acceptable, observation may be more appropriate

Table 7.1 Examples of the type of question, approach, method and data produced

Question	Approach	Method	Data
How much, many, often, what do people think, believe, how well are we doing? (Level 1)	Descriptive quantitative survey, audit.	Observation, questionnaires, interviews, documents	Numeric
What is the lived experience, how do people behave, interpret situations? (Level 1)	Descriptive, qualitative, phenomenological, ethnographic	In-depth interviews, observation, documentary accounts (diaries, etc.)	Words in the form of dialogue, quotes, observation
Which variable is related to another, or series of others? Does this method correlate with a better outcome than another? (Level 2)	Correlation survey, physiological measurement Quasi-experimental	Physiological tests, measurement scales, questionnaires, interviews observation, documents	Numeric
Is this method better than an alternative? Is there a cause and effect relationship between an independent and dependent variable? (Level 3)	Randomised control trial	Physiological tests, measurement scales, questionnaires, interviews observation, documents	Numeric

than depending on memory or the provision of complex details through interviews or questionnaires. A level-three question will usually make it clear that an experimental design will be needed because it involves decisions on what is more effective, appropriate or successful. The question will also suggest the type of data to be collected. In the main, this will relate to whether quantitative data in the form of numbers will be gathered, or whether qualitative data in the form of words will be necessary.

CONSTRUCTING A RESEARCH QUESTION

How do we construct a research question? Questions can take an *interrogative* or a *declarative* form. The interrogative form is written in exactly the same way as a question. For example, 'What influences women to continue breastfeeding for longer than 4 weeks?' The second, declarative form is used more often in research reports, and is a statement of the purpose of the study. This identifies what particular event, phenomenon or situation the study is to consider and usually starts with such statements as:

- to examine,
- to identify,
- to describe,
- to explore.

Table 7.2 *Examples of research aims*

Author	Aim	Level
Sweet and Darbyshire (2009)	To explore fathers' experiences of the breastfeeding of their very-low-birthweight preterm babies from birth to 12 months of age. (Qualitative)	1
Lindgren et al. (2010)	To describe women's self-reported perceptions of risk related to childbirth ahead of their planned home birth and the strategies for managing these perceived risks. (Quantitative Survey)	1
Kerrigan and Kingdom (2010)	To establish the incidence of obesity in the pregnant population in a large city in the North West of England, identify links between obesity and social deprivation, and compare outcomes of pregnancy in obese and non-obese women. (Quantitative Correlation)	2
McDonald et al. (2010)	To evaluate the effects of an extended midwifery support (EMS) programme on the proportion of women who breast feed fully to 6 months. (Quantitative Randomised Control Trial)	3

An example would be 'to identify some of the factors that influence woman to breastfeed for longer than 4 weeks'.

The statement of the aim should allow the reader to picture what will happen to whom in a study. This means there should be an indication of what information or variable is to be gathered or examined, perhaps in relation to another variable, and from whom or what this information will be collected, that is, the sample involved in the study. Table 7.2 illustrates some examples of research aims written in this style.

Precisely worded research questions will provide more direction and clarity for a study. However, although the researcher may start with a clear statement of the research problem, it is important to examine the literature carefully to establish what is known already about the topic. In particular, the researcher should search for known possible relationships between the variables in the study. At this stage the researcher should examine the way similar studies have framed their questions, and the way in which they have provided concept definitions and operational definitions for variables, as these may be useful in developing a new study.

THE HYPOTHESIS

In level-two and -three questions, the researcher may state a *hypothesis*. This can be defined as the prediction the researcher makes at the beginning of the study that links an independent variable to a dependent variable. As level-one questions have only one variable, we can see why they do not require a hypothesis. A further definition of the hypothesis is provided by Polit and Beck (2008: 66) as follows:

A hypothesis is a statement of the researcher's expectations about relationships between study variables. Hypotheses, in other words, are predictions of expected outcomes; they state the relationships researchers expect to find as a result of the study.

The purpose of the hypothesis is to provide a means of demonstrating whether the researcher's prediction or 'hunch' can be accepted or rejected. Researchers do not say that a hypothesis has been *proved* or *disproved*, as it is difficult to be that certain since research always includes a margin of error. From the researcher's point of view, a hypothesis gives the study direction, as the design must take into account how the variables will be measured and the statistical approach to testing the results to see if a relationship between the variables can be demonstrated. Thus, Polit and Beck (2008: 94) suggest that hypotheses force the researcher to think logically and to exercise critical judgement by considering the study within the context of current knowledge and literature. They also believe that stating a hypothesis helps avoid superficiality by challenging the researcher to consider outcomes at the start of a study, and not simply come up with a possible explanation to fit findings where one has not been constructed.

The hypothesis can take one of the following forms:

- directional or 'one-tailed' hypothesis,
- non-directional or 'two-tailed hypothesis,
- null-hypothesis.

DIRECTIONAL OR 'ONE-TAILED' HYPOTHESIS

Here, a prediction is made about the likely outcome between two variables, e.g. *'women who deliver in a midwifery-led unit will be discharged quicker than those on consultant-led units'*. In this case, the dependent variable is the length of time between the birth and discharge home, and the independent variable is the form of care, i.e. midwifery-led or consultant-led. There is a directional, or *'one-tailed hypothesis'*, because we have predicted the results will be *more than* or *less than* that found in a comparable situation, that is, we have predicted the direction of the result. A study with this kind of hypothesis could be a level-two question where we are comparing a group of women under midwifery-led care and with a group under consultant-led care and looking for correlation or pattern between the time period between the birth and discharge home and level of intervention, or it could be experimental where we randomly allocate women to either a midwifery-led unit or consultant-led unit and the outcome measure would be the time between birth and discharge. In this case it would be a level-three question, as we would be deliberately manipulating the independent variable –the form of care – and looking for a more explicit cause-and-effect relationship with the outcome – the time from birth to discharge.

NON-DIRECTIONAL OR 'TWO-TAILED' HYPOTHESIS

With a non-directional hypothesis, although a prediction is made, it is not stated in which direction the outcome will be more favourable, e.g. *'there will* be a difference in the length of time between birth and discharge home in those women who deliver in a midwifery-led unit in comparison with those who deliver in a consultant-led unit'. In this example it could be that those gave birth in the midwifery-led unit will a longer length of time before going home, or vice versa. All that is predicted is that there will be a difference. This form is called a *two-tailed hypothesis*, as the result could go in either of two directions (or tails). A non-directional hypothesis would be used where the researcher feels there is an association, or pattern, but is uncertain of the exact nature, and so keeps the direction of the findings open.

NULL-HYPOTHESIS

A null-hypothesis follows the convention in experiments where the researcher demonstrates an absence of bias by stating that he or she does not expect to find a difference between the two groups in the study, e.g. *'there will be no difference in the length of time between the birth and discharge home between those women who deliver in a midwifery-led unit or those who delivery in a consultant-led unit'*. The null-hypothesis is known as the hypothesis of no difference and is related to statistical convention where, if a difference is found, then the null-hypothesis (that there is no difference) has to be rejected. In other words, it has been demonstrated that there is a difference between the groups included in the study.

The null-hypothesis is known as the *statistical hypothesis*, as the aim is to establish statistically whether there is sufficient evidence to accept or reject it. If the statistical hypothesis is rejected, then its opposite, the scientific or *research hypothesis*, is accepted. The statistical hypothesis and the research hypothesis are different sides of the same coin, where, in reality, one cannot exist without the existence of the other, its opposite. Which one is 'face-up', or currently accepted, depends on the strength of the statistical evidence to support it. The research hypothesis is another name for the first two examples of the hypothesis examined above, that is, the directional or non-directional hypothesis.

Not all experimental research states a hypothesis; where they are provided, medical research tends to use the null-hypothesis form and midwifery and nursing research tend to use the research hypothesis and suggest the direction of the outcome.

COMPLEX HYPOTHESES

This form of the hypothesis is very similar to the simple hypothesis except there is more than one dependent variable, e.g. women who give birth in a midwifery-led unit will have a lower level of intervention during the birth and a lower level of analgesia than those who give birth in a consultant-led unit. It is more usual to see hypotheses expressed separately as two simple hypotheses, as this makes them easy to test and understand.

An example of a complex hypothesis is the following by Svensson et al. (2009: 116) who carried out a randomised control trial on two antenatal education programmes for first-time parents in Sydney, Australia. See if you can identify the dependent variables in the following:

Women who attended the 'Having a Baby' programme would have higher perceived parenting self-efficacy and knowledge scores, and lower baby worry scores 8 weeks after the birth compared with those who attended the regular programme.

In this example the outcome measure, or dependent variables (see Chapter 2) are 'parenting self-efficacy,' 'knowledge' and 'baby worries'. Each of these will form a variable in the study that will need to be clearly defined and operationalised (measured) using some kind of scoring system. The independent variable (see Chapter 2) would be the form of antenatal education.

It is more usual to see the dependent variables listed separately in a number of hypotheses, as it increases clarity if the results demonstrate that some are rejected and some are accepted.

CONDUCTING RESEARCH

For those undertaking research, the development of the research question is one of the most important steps in the research process. The preliminary stages involve ensuring that a problem area is suitable for research. This concerns the relevance of the topic. It is also important to check that the study is feasible in terms of access to the sample, the resources required to carry out the study, the ethical implications, cooperation from key people involved, and the skills of the researcher, as well as the availability of sufficient time to complete the research.

A thorough review of the literature is crucial, as this will provide valuable background information on the topic, including the possible relationships between variables that might already have been discovered. It is also useful for discovering the way other authors have developed concept and operational definitions for the variables. The literature will help the researcher decide on an appropriate level of question. The methods used in previous studies, including the way the data have been analysed, will also influence the design.

The statement of the research question should be clear. The researcher must be confident that it is possible to answer the research question through data collection. The question should make reference to the sample from whom the data will be gathered, and where there is more than one variable, the nature of any relationships should be made clear.

If the level of the question is level two or three, then a hypothesis may be constructed to demonstrate the prediction to be tested through data collection, and whether an association is being considered, or a cause-and-effect relationship.

Once the research question has been constructed, along with the hypothesis if appropriate, it is worth asking, 'Will the information I am collecting allow me to answer the aim?' The final check is to ensure that the research question is not too large to be undertaken in its entirety. Would it be better to take on only one aspect of this problem area and leave the larger questions either to a future project or to someone else?

CRITIQUING RESEARCH

The research question is pivotal to critiquing a research article. This is because so many decisions follow as a consequence of the question wording. The level of the question, for instance, dictates whether the design should be descriptive, correlative or experimental. It is important that the researcher is consistent in the design, which should flow from the aim.

The location of the aim is usually in the abstract under the title in those journals that provide one. It is also commonly found just above the subheading 'method' following the review of the literature in the main body of a research article. Look for the phrase 'the aim of the research was to ...'; the words stating with '*to*' will form the aim or terms of reference.

If the question is level two or three, there may be a hypothesis, although many researchers omit this. Where a hypothesis is stated, is it directional, non-directional, or a null-hypothesis? Does it indicate a relationship between an independent and dependent variable in a named sample, and is the nature of that relationship stated? Is the researcher looking for an association, or a cause-and-effect relationship between the variables? If it is the latter, then the study should be experimental and the researcher should be responsible for introducing the independent variable.

Whether we are dealing with one or several variables, in quantitative research the researcher should provide concept and operational definitions for each one identified in the aim or hypotheses. Are these clear and unambiguous?

Finally, at the end of the research article, consider whether the researcher has clearly answered the aim? Is there a clear conclusion that relates to and echoes the way the aim was worded? Where the researcher stated one or more hypothesis, is there a clear statement as to whether each of these has been accepted or rejected? Most importantly, given the results of the research, do you feel the aim has been adequately answered?

KEY POINTS

- Research studies revolve around collecting information to answer the study aim or research question.
- The way these are constructed will influence the level of the question and the way the study is constructed.
- Research questions must be capable of being answered; they must be feasible and above all relevant to practice or service delivery.
- Level-two and- three questions may have a stated hypothesis that provides an indication of the prediction the researcher is making between the variables in the study.

REFERENCES

Atkinson, I., 2008. Asking research questions. In: Watson, R., McKenna, H., Cowman, S., Keady, J. (Eds.), Nursing Research: Designs and Methods. Churchill Livingstone, Edinburgh.

Burns, N., Grove, S., 2009. The Practice of Nursing Research: Appraisal, Synthesis, and Generation of Evidence. sixth ed. Saunders, St Louis.

Houser, J., 2008. Nursing Research: Reading, Using and Creating Evidence. Jones and Bartlett, Sudbury.

Kerrigan, A., Kingdom, C., 2010. Maternal obesity and pregnancy: a retrospective study. Midwifery 26 (1), 138–146.

Lindgren, H., Rådestad, I., Christensson, K., Wally-Bystrom, K., Hildingsson, I., 2010. Perceptions of risk and risk management among 735 women who opted for a home birth. Midwifery 26 (2), 163–172.

McDonald, S., Henderson, J., Faulkner, S., Evans, S., Hagen, R., 2010. Effect of an extended midwifery postnatal support programme on the duration of breast feeding: A randomised controlled trial. Midwifery 26 (1), 88–100.

Polit, D., Beck, C., 2008. Nursing Research: Generating and Assessing Evidence for Nursing Practice. eighth ed. Lippincott Williams and Wilkins, Philadelphia.

Svensson, J., Barclay, L., Cooke, M., 2009. Randomised-controlled trial of two antenatal education programmes. Midwifery 25 (2), 114–125.

Sweet, L., Darbyshire, P., 2009. Fathers and breast feeding very-low-birthweight preterm babies. Midwifery 25 (5), 540–553.

Wood, M., Ross-Kerr, J., 2006. Basic Steps in Planning Nursing Research: From Question to Proposal. sixth ed. Jones and Bartlett, Sudbury.

Ethics and research

Research is not simply about the process of data collection; it is also concerned with the conduct of the researcher and the manner in which a study is carried out. Under research governance, this has to conform to set standards in the relationship between the researcher and those participating in the research, and the ethical management of the whole project. As with clinical practice, ethics in research must illustrate respect and maintain the trust that people have in health professionals, health organisations and researchers.

Ethical issues are a particular concern where research involves vulnerable groups such as women in pregnancy and labour, and babies, who form an even more vulnerable group. Both need their human rights respected and their safety and privacy safeguarded. Midwives work under the midwifery rules (**NMC 2004**) and a professional code of conduct (**NMC 2008**), and it is right that midwives are accountable for the way in which they conduct themselves when carrying out research. In the **UK** they must conform to the guidelines laid down in the *Research Governance Framework for Health and Social Care* (**DoH 2005**).

This chapter will examine the ethical issues raised by research in maternity services. These relate to the protection of fundamental human rights, and the obligations and responsibilities of the researcher in carrying out research. The main issues covered include informed consent, confidentiality, justice, and an assessment of possible benefits of participation in research balanced against possible disadvantages or 'harm'.

Ethics can be defined as a code of behaviour considered correct, or, as Houser (2008: 53) puts it, 'the study of right and wrong'. Within a research context, the Economic and Social Research Council (ESRC) (2010: 40) give the following definition:

> *Research Ethics refers to the moral principles guiding research, from its inception through to completion and publication of results and beyond – for example, the curation [safekeeping] of data and physical samples after the research has been published.*

© 2011 Elsevier Ltd. All rights reserved.

Ethics control what is permissible within research, making it is impossible to plan research in health care without anticipating and solving the ethical issues it raises. The increasing complexity and sophistication of research means that ethical issues have become more central to discussions about research than ever before (Bryman 2008). This has been reinforced by one high-profile example of participants in research suffering organ failure and serious illness as a result of inclusion in a drug trial (Mayor 2006, Wood and Darbyshire 2006) and researcher misconduct where fictitious studies have been report in journals (Smith 2006). These have justified the continual attempts to make the safety and human respect of those receiving care paramount. Ethics are now the part of the research process that the researcher has to get right; otherwise the study will not get approval to take place.

Ethics relate to two groups of people; those carrying out research, who should be aware of their obligations and responsibilities in the way in which they carry out their activities, and the 'researched upon', who have basic human rights that should be protected. As with ethics generally, those relating to research provide a basis for deciding whether certain behaviour can be regarded as acceptable according to agreed principles and values. There are a number of problems implicit in this, as different people may have conflicting views and values on what is acceptable. To overcome this dilemma, Local Research Ethics Committees (LRECs) operate to consider research projects at a planning stage to ensure that they conform to national ethical guidelines and standards.

As medical research has been carried out for far longer and is more frequently conducted than midwifery research, it is not surprising that ethical principles have been developed with medical research very much in mind. This means that ethics committees often use the experimental approach synonymous with the 'scientific' method as the 'gold standard' against which others are measured. Ethical issues are therefore considered very much in relation to the potentially more dangerous implications of clinical trials.

Is it important for all midwives to know about research ethics? The simple answer is 'yes'. Firstly, in making practice research-based the ethical aspects of a study must also be judged. It is not morally safe to implement research if it does not conform to ethical principles, as it casts doubt on the researcher's honesty and integrity concerning all aspects of the study. Secondly, knowledge of research ethics may also be crucial if the midwife has to act as advocate for an individual mother, baby and family. This may include situations where someone has been invited to take part in research that is not ethical. The RCN (2007) guidelines on research, which have been adopted by midwifery, also point out that nurses and midwives may be called upon to act as witnesses to ensure that free and informed consent has been given prior to involvement in research. Under these circumstances, the midwife must be satisfied that the person concerned has received relevant information to make an informed decision, and is not under any duress or coercion to participate. What actually constitutes coercion can be difficult to identify but Johnson and Long's (2010) explanation is helpful in that they suggest it is the use of 'undue pressure or leverage', such as an existing relationship with someone that will influence them to take part in a study. So, a midwife approaching those for whom they have already given care and advice may be seen to be coercing them to take part as they may feel that an obligation already exists and so the freedom to say 'no' is reduced in such cases.

What, then, comes under the heading of ethical issues in research? According to the RCN (2007: 3) the essential elements that must be observed by all researchers include:

- informed consent,
- confidentiality,
- data protection,
- right to withdraw,
- potential benefits and the potential harms.

These will be covered throughout this chapter. The next section summarises the more recent development of ethics within health care.

BOX 8.1 Major international ethical codes

The Nuremberg code
This was developed in 1947 as a result of the human experimentation carried out by the Nazi regime during World War II. The code consists of 10 principles that have been influential in the conduct of research, particularly experimental research, throughout the world. The major principle relates to obtaining informed consent from those involved in research. Although the code relates to physical interventions, account is also taken of psychological and emotional harm. One criticism of the code is that it depends on self-regulation by the experimenter.

The declaration of Helsinki
These guidelines were developed by the World Medical Assembly (WMA) in Finland in 1964 and updated regularly since then, including October 2008 (available at http://www.wma.net/en/30publications/10policies/b3/index.html). In addition to re-emphasising the principles of the Nuremberg Code, it developed clauses to protect subjects' human rights. An important distinction is made between therapeutic and non-therapeutic research. Therapeutic research relates to situations where the individual may potentially benefit physically from the research, whereas in non-therapeutic research subjects probably will not benefit physically, although others may benefit in the future.

The Belmont report
The Belmont Report of 1978 highlighted what has become the three basic ethical principles of research:
1. respect for persons,
2. beneficence,
3. justice.

One of the report's aims was to develop guidelines on the selection of those included in the research. The report emphasises the need for written consent of subjects, and the obligation of the researcher to assess the possible risk and benefits related to participation in research.

HISTORICAL DEVELOPMENT OF ETHICAL PRINCIPLES

The present guidelines on research ethics have been influenced by a number of internationally accepted codes on the conduct of research. These were developed following the revelation of a number of scientific experiments on humans that were clearly unethical. Following their revelation, it was agreed that society should be protected from anyone who might carry out research that leads to the death or injury of those taking part. Through a series of refinements, the codes outlined in Box 8.1 have influenced present-day research practice in all branches of health care.

NURSING AND MIDWIFERY GUIDELINES

Ethical guidelines for nursing research were developed much later than those in medicine. The American Nurses' Association (ANA) developed their principles in 1968, and have updated them periodically. These cover not only the basic principles regarding the use of human subjects, but also the role of the nurse as researcher and practitioner. In Britain, guidelines were produced by the RCN in 1977 with an update in 2007 (RCN 2007). This reinforces the major ethical issues regarding health care research and provides guidance on research governance, as explained below. The guideline provides helpful links to all the sources of information needed to apply for ethical approval. No separate guidelines exist for midwifery.

RESEARCH GOVERNANCE

Since 2005, research governance has been a core standard for all organisations delivering NHS care (DoH 2005) and illustrates the importance on the management of research activity in the UK as well as the USA, Canada and Australia. Haig (2008: 125) offers the following definition of clinical governance:

> *Research governance is a framework through which institutions are accountable for ethical quality, scientific acceptability and management of participant safety in research that they sponsor or permit.*

Its role is to make organisations accountable for high standards in the protection of those participating in research. The intension is to increase the quality of research and to ensure that it is 'managed' safely and effectively. The DoH (2005) clinical governance framework is summarised under the following headings, using some of the original wording:

1. ETHICS

All research involving patients, service users, care professionals or volunteers, or their organs, tissue or data, must be reviewed independently to ensure it meets ethical standards. This is achieved through a local research ethics committee (LREC), or equivalent within higher education. The study design must illustrate the high priority given to safeguarding the dignity, rights, safety and well-being of participants in a study. Informed consent is at the heart of ethical research and relates to staff as well as those receiving health care. Data collected, particularly from patients, should be used appropriately and protected. Secure systems must protect confidential information. Relevant service users and carers or their representative groups should be involved wherever possible in the design, conduct, analysis and reporting of research. Those included in research studies should reflect the diversity of groups within society. Risks, pain or discomfort to the individual must be minimised, but where they do exist, any risks must be in proportion to the potential benefit to the participant.

2. SCIENCE

Any research proposal must demonstrate a thorough search of current sources of knowledge has taken place to ensure that answers sought do not already exist. This is to avoid needless duplication of effort. The methodological details of any study must be examined by experts to ensure that the study is sound. There are special procedures for assessing the standard of clinical trials involving the testing of medicines and studies using human embryos. Data collected must be kept for an appropriate time for further use and monitoring.

3. INFORMATION

There should be free public access to information on studies that are being conducted and on their results once complete, whether the outcomes were favourable or not. In particularly, those involved in a study should have access to the findings along with those who could benefit from them. Studies should be open to critical review through scientific and professional channels. Researchers are under an obligation at the planning stage to state how they will disseminate the results of their study. This is to ensure that potential benefits from new knowledge are not lost by not publishing the results, or not making them available to key people and organisations.

4. HEALTH, SAFETY AND EMPLOYMENT

Research involving potentially dangerous or harmful equipment, substances or organisms should give priority to the safety of participants and other staff at all times, and health and safety regulations must be strictly observed. This should include the provision of information, containment, shielding and monitoring as required. In midwifery, the personal safety of the researcher where research is undertaken in someone's home must be protected and built into the method of data collection.

5. FINANCE AND INTELLECTUAL PROPERTY

Researchers and the organisations or departments in which they work should demonstrate financial honesty in the use of public funds by following appropriate financial procedures. They must also demonstrate they have funding to pay for compensation in the event of any negligent harm to those taking part in studies. The intellectual property rights of those carrying out the study should also be protected.

As ethics are not static, these guidelines may be revised to match the changes in research approaches and the ethical issues raised by them. For example, ethical guidelines may change with the increased collection of data through the internet and the implications this has for confidentially, informed consent and privacy (Eynon et al. 2008).

In summary, clinical governance is an attempt to control and 'manage' research and achieve high standards through the involvement of 'sponsors' such as local health boards who are accountable for the conduct of researchers and research teams who work within them. Thus, the intention is the continuing production of high-quality research that can have a real impact on health care through the application of research knowledge to practice.

LOCAL RESEARCH ETHICS COMMITTEES

The main body involved in assessing the ethical viability of research proposals in the UK is a local research ethics committee (LREC). It is important to emphasise that LRECs are concerned with research and not audit or service evaluation. However, both audit and service evaluation should be carried out in an ethical, honest and accurate way.

Who sits on an LREC? The recommended membership of LRECs is a maximum of 18 members covering a broad range of experience and expertise, so that the scientific, clinical and methodological aspects of a research proposal can be considered (Parliamentary Office of Science Technology 2005). They should include both sexes and a wide age range and a mixture of 'expert' and 'lay' members. At least one-third should be lay members who are independent of the NHS. At least half of the lay members should be people who have never been health professionals and who have never been involved in carrying out research involving human participants.

In the United States, the counterpart of the LREC is the institutional review board (IRB). This is required to have at least five members from various backgrounds, who reflect professional, gender, racial and cultural diversity. If a research study centres on vulnerable subjects, the IRB should also include members with knowledge about and experience of this group. Membership must include one member whose concerns are non-scientific, such as a lawyer, member of the clergy and at least one member from outside the health organisation. The role of the IRB, as with the LREC, is to protect the human rights of those involved in research (Burns and Grove 2009).

ETHICAL PRINCIPLES CONCERNING BASIC HUMAN RIGHTS

According to the DoH (2005: 7) Research Governance Framework, the dignity, rights, safety and well-being of participants must be the primary consideration in any research study. These are highlighted and addressed through ethical principles relating to human rights. In this section the three basic human rights of *respect for individual autonomy, protection from harm* and *justice* will be examined. These principles are presented in Table 8.1, which outlines for each

Table 8.1 *Issues involved in achieving an ethical study*

Basic human principle involved	Achieved through	Denied by
Respect for individual autonomy	Informed consent	Right to refuse to participate or to withdraw at any point not explained
Lack of clear written information on the study given to subjects
Comprehension of information not checked
Confidentiality and anonymity not assured
Coerced to participate
Excessive or unrealistic rewards promised
Deception regarding study details
Existing relationship between researchers and subjects exploited
Covert data collection
Protection of participants (beneficence/non-maleficence)	Risk versus benefit ratio	Risks outweigh benefits
Unacceptable level of pain, discomfort or distress
Confidentiality and anonymity not protected
Access to original data not safeguarded
No debriefing provided or referral to appropriate agencies offered where appropriate
Justice	Fair selection of sample	Only vulnerable or disadvantaged group included
Captive group used, or coerced, with no opportunity to refuse or withdraw without application of sanction

of the principles how the researcher demonstrates it has been achieved, and, just as importantly, some of the elements that would suggest that the basic human rights have been denied.

RESPECT FOR INDIVIDUAL AUTONOMY

This is based on the ethical principle that individuals have the right to make decisions about themselves and their life and so be 'self-governing' or *autonomous*. Individuals should be asked if they would like to take part in research on the understanding that they have the right to refuse or, if they accept, can withdraw from the research at any time without any adverse consequences for the care they receive. This principle of autonomy is a familiar concept in midwifery, where women are encouraged through empowerment to have control over decisions affecting them. Similarly, it is not for others to decide if someone should or should not take part in research; only the individual (or in the case of babies, a parent) is in a position to make that decision.

How is respect for individual autonomy achieved? Table 8.1 illustrates that this principle is achieved through informed consent, also called *'valid consent'* (ESRC 2010). According to the Research Governance Framework (DoH 2005) informed consent is at the heart of ethical research. However, this is not a simple matter of someone saying 'yes I will take part in this study'. The important word is *'informed'* consent. For this to be achieved, the following should be evident:

- full disclosure of details about the study,
- a statement that there is no obligation to take part, and that there are no consequences if the decision to participate is 'no',
- assurance that the individual can withdraw at any time without any negative consequences,
- confirmation of confidentiality and anonymity,
- care that all the information concerning involvement is understood,
- meaningful provision of the opportunity to ask questions,
- absence of pressure, unfair inducements or coercion to take part.

What should the researcher tell a prospective subject in a study before we can say that a decision to participate was informed or valid? A good way of answering this is to imagine that someone approaches you and asks if you would take part in their research. What information would you want to know before you said 'yes'?

Your answer might be quite a long list, including who the people were; what organisation they represented; what taking part would involve, particularly if there is anything invasive, painful, risky or embarrassing; the aim of the project; what will happen to the information gathered and who might have access to that information. Anyone participating in research has the right to expect all of these questions to be answered if autonomy is to be protected. The researcher must ensure that all the details included in Box 8.2 are covered and given to anyone taking part in a study in an information sheet before they can claim that informed consent has been achieved.

Gaining consent is not simply a matter of giving information; it should be given in words and a language that the individual can understand. This relates to the principle of comprehension. In some instances, a judgement may have to be made on the educational competence of the individual to understand the information and the implications of it, or whether they have the metal capacity to make a judgement as outlined in the Mental Capacity Act 2005 (Dept. of Constitutional Affairs 2007).

BOX 8.2 Information required to achieve informed consent

The identification of the researcher and their organisation
The purpose of the study
Potential participants informed they need not volunteer
Assured they have the right to withdraw at any time
The nature of the participation (what will happen over what period of time)
Possible risks or implications of participating, and any anticipated benefits
Assurance of confidentiality
Offered the opportunity to ask questions and time to consider the invitation

In midwifery, the timing and circumstances under which consent is gained is crucial. It is accepted that women should not be recruited into studies when they are in labour, as they are very vulnerable. This is because they may have difficulty in concentrating on the details of a request to participate in a research study when they are experiencing contractions, anxious about the birth, and possibly experiencing the effects of analgesia (Vernon et al. 2006). The principle is that women should be asked to participate in research during pregnancy and not during labour.

Consideration has also to be given to gaining written consent. The DoH (2005) suggests that written consent should be obtained following receipt of a clearly written information sheet explaining the nature of the study. People should then be given a reasonable period of time to consider whether to participate or not. It is this last issue that is problematic if women are asked to participate once in labour, as it allows no time for consideration or reflection.

Confidentiality and anonymity

A vital component of informed consent is the assurance of confidentiality and anonymity. Confidentiality is a basic ethical principle used in many professional settings, such as the law and the church and relates to the researcher ensuring that unauthorised people do not have access to the raw data collected in the research (Burns and Grove 2009). Anonymity means that steps are taken to protect the identity of an individual by neither giving their name when presenting research results, nor including identifying details that might reveal their identity. This might include such things as personal characteristics or the name of work areas where it may be possible to deduce, with reasonable accuracy, the identity of the individual.

Confidentiality does not mean that the information will not be shared with others, as research findings frequently include verbal comments from respondents; the key is that the person cannot be identified, and so remains anonymous.

The main issue is that of data security to ensure that others do not have access to the raw data (Wood and Ross-Kerr 2006). This involves the researcher storing the data in such a way that no unauthorised person can gain access to it. This applies not only to paper copies of information but also raw data containing names or identifying details kept on a computer. Here the researcher must follow the principles of the Data Protection Act 1998. This involves the right of individuals to see the information that is kept on them, and their right not to have that information passed on to another party.

AVOIDING HARM

The second ethical principle is that of minimising harm. This is discussed in the literature under a number of different headings and can be referred to as the protection of subjects, or *beneficence* and *nonmaleficence* (terms that are useful to use with an explanation in any course work). Holloway and Wheeler (2010) define beneficence as providing benefits and balancing benefits against risks and costs, while nonmaleficence, they suggest, is avoiding causing harm to individuals. These are similar concepts to those in most professional codes of conduct; here, the researcher has an obligation to protect the rights and well-being of those involved in research.

The main categories of risk are physical, psychological and emotional, although Burns and Grove (2009) add they can also be social and economic. Although midwifery researchers are not likely to set out to inflict harm, it should be acknowledged that some form of harm or discomfort might be a consequence of participating in a study (Johnson and Long 2010). For example, some procedures are uncomfortable or result in some pain. However, this is unlikely to be lasting or cause permanent damage. To some extent, all research involves some risks, but in most cases the risk is minimal and no greater than those commonly encountered in our daily life, or routinely experienced during physical or psychological tests and procedures. However, the researcher must carry out a risk assessment of the type, severity and likelihood of harm in a study, and the extent of any risk should be discussed with those taking part before they enter into a study.

The protection of the individual from harm applies equally to psychological or emotional distress as well as physical consequences. This can occur not only during research involving clinical intervention, but also in surveys involving questionnaires or interviews. This may also be applied to qualitative research involving interviews or observation. These may entail an element of intrusion, embarrassment or, in some cases, such as describing a negative birth experience or the loss of a baby, a high degree of emotional distress and pain, as well as anxiety or guilt. Under these circumstances the researcher must weigh up the costs to the individual very carefully.

This does not mean that such studies should not be undertaken, as they may benefit others through a greater understanding of the experiences described. However, it does emphasise the need for the researcher to be sensitive to this element of harm. Where an individual is distressed, it will involve identifying whether, in the person's own interests, the researcher should call a halt to an interview or clinical procedure, for example. It also means that individuals should be told beforehand that there might be a possibility of painful memories arising during the course of the study. If there is a likelihood of emotional distress, then the researcher must be in a position to counsel the individual, or arrange with counselling agencies to accept referrals should the need arise. It is these kinds of details that ethics committees would expect to see in the outline of intended research projects.

JUSTICE

Justice, the third and final principle, can be overlooked at the planning stage, because of the focus on the previous ethical issues. However, it is just as important, as it relates to the fair treatment and the equal distribution of benefit and burden amongst those in the study (Houser 2008). In selecting the study population, the researcher should ensure that the sampling is inclusive and those chosen represent the diversity of society in regard to major groups (Johnson and Long 2010). This would meet Polit and Beck's (2008) criteria of justice, which implies fairness and equity for those who may benefit

In addition to a LREC, the research proposal may need to be seen by a local research and development (R&D) unit which will assess and give advice on the technical or methodological aspects. Support should also be gained from managers, relevant clinicians and any other 'gatekeepers' involved in accessing individuals or data. It is always wise to insist on written confirmation of support when others are involved, in case key people 'move on' prior to or during the study.

Permission to start a study is one of the most important steps in the research process. There can be considerable delays and disappointment if this does not go smoothly. Do everything you can to ensure that the ethical and methodological sections of your research proposal reach a high standard, and that these are based on sound knowledge and the principles laid down in the most recent clinical governance guidelines.

CRITIQUING RESEARCH

To some extent when it comes to critiquing this aspect of the research process, midwives already have some knowledge and experience to draw on. Indeed, Kinnane (2009) suggests that ethics are embedded in every encounter a midwife has, and so it is a case of applying this knowledge to the evaluation of the ethical issues raised by studies, and the way in which they were resolved by the researcher.

Although an author may mention some ethical issues in a report, there is not always space to cover all the aspects covered in this chapter. This means that only brief mention may be made of the approval by an ethics committee, the gaining of informed consent, and the assurances of confidentiality or anonymity. Often, the reader is left to assume that things have been carefully thought out and ethical safeguards applied. Indeed, Johnson and Long (2010) regret the lack of detail included in many studies that allow judgements on the ethical dimension.

It is reasonable for the reader to ask the following questions as a minimum:

- Was the study submitted to an ethics committee (LREC)? In the case of an American study, is there mention of an institutional review board (IRB)?
- Is there evidence of freedom from bias in the way the researcher conducted the study? In particular, did anybody or organisation that might have had a vested interest in a positive outcome sponsor the author(s)?
- Was informed consent gained?
- Were there any risks of discomfort or distress involved in taking part in the study not anticipated by the researcher, or not justified by the likely benefits to the individual/others in a similar situation?
- Did the researcher conduct the research in a sensitive manner in regard to the wording of questions and privacy afforded individuals?
- Were any foreseeable discomforts, side effects or potential risks outlined to subjects before they gave informed consent?
- Was a pilot study undertaken that may have identified any risks to the individual?

KEY POINTS

- Research is not simply a process of gathering data; it also involves ethical issues in conducting the study.
- Ethics relate to the protection of the human rights of those involved in research, and the obligations and responsibilities of the researcher. The main human rights the researcher must illustrate are respect for the individual, the protection against harm, and justice (fair treatment).
- Informed consent relates to the extent to which an individual agrees to take part in a study on the basis of a clear understanding of the purpose of the research and the implications of agreeing to take part.
- The 'harm versus benefits' ratio is an attempt to weigh up the possible disadvantages for an individual taking part in a study against the possible positive effects either for them or others in the future.
- Justice relates to the fair treatment of all those who are potentially or actually involved in the research process.
- All health research should be approved by a local research ethics committee (LREC) whose role is to protect the public and health staff against harm and exploitation. There may also be a local research and development (R&D) unit that will examine the technical aspects of a study prior to it going to an ethics committee.
- Projects that can be classified as audit or service evaluation are not required to be assessed by an ethics committee, but those responsible should still be mindful of the way the information is collected and the use to which it is put.

REFERENCES

Bryman, A., 2008. Social Research Methods, third ed. Oxford University Press, Oxford.

Burns, N., Grove, S., 2009. The Practice of Nursing Research: Appraisal, Synthesis, and Generation of Evidence, sixth ed. Saunders, St Louis.

Department of Constitutional Affairs, 2007. Mental Capacity Act 2005. www.opsi.gov.uk/acts/acts2005/related/ukpgacop_20050009_en.pdf (accessed 24.04.10.).

DoH, 2005. Research Governance Framework for Health and Social Care, second ed. DoH, London.

Economic and Social Research Council (ESRC), 2010. Framework for Research Ethics. http://www.esrcsocietytoday.ac.uk/ESRCInfoCentre/Images/Framework%20for%20Research%20Ethics%202010_tcm6-35811.pdf (accessed: 23.04.10.).

Eynon, R., Fry, J., Schroeder, R., 2008. The ethics of internet research. In: Fielding, N., Lee, R., Blank, G. (Eds.), The Sage Handbook of Online Research Methods. Sage, London.

Haig, C., 2008. Research governance and research ethics. In: Watson, R., McKenna, H., Cowman, S., Keady, J. (Eds.), Nursing Research: Designs and Methods. Edinburgh, Churchill Livingstone.

Holloway, I., Wheeler, S., 2010. Qualitative Research for Nurses, third ed. Wiley-Blackwell, Chichester.

Houser, J., 2008. Nursing Research: Reading, Using and Creating Evidence. Jones and Bartlett, Sudbury.

Johnson, M., Long, T., 2010. Research ethics. In: Gerrish, K., Lacey, A. (Eds.), The Research Process in Nursing, sixth ed. Wiley-Blackwell, Chichester.

Kinnane, J., 2009. Ethics on-the-run. British Journal of Midwifery 17 (1), 30–35.

Mayor, S., 2006. Severe adverse reactions prompt call for trial design changes. Br. Med. J. 332 (7543), 683.

NMC, 2004. Midwives Rules and Standards. NMC, London.

NMC, 2008. The Code: Standards of conduct, performance and ethics for nurses and midwives. NMC, London.

Parliamentary Office of Science and Technology (POST), 2005. Postnote Number 243: Ethical Scrutiny of Research. www.parliament.uk/documents/upload/postpn243.pdf (accessed 23.04.10.).

Polit, D., Beck, C., 2008. Nursing Research: Generating and Assessing Evidence for Nursing Practice, eighth ed. Lippincott Williams and Wilkins, Philadelphia.

Royal College of Nursing (RCN), 2007. Research Ethics: RCN Guidelines for Nurses. RCN, London.

Smith, R., 2006. Research misconduct: the poisoning of the well. J. R. Soc. Med. 99 (5), 232–237.

Vernon, G., Alfirevic, Z., Weeks, A., 2006. Issues of informed consent for intrapartum trials: a suggested consent pathway from the experience of the Release trial. Trials Journal http://www.trialsjournal.com/content/pdf/1745-6215-7-13.pdf (accessed 23.04.10.).

Wood, A., Darbyshire, J., 2006. Injury to research volunteers – the clinical-research nightmare. N. Engl. J. Med. 354 (18), 1869–1871.

Wood, M., Ross-Kerr, J., 2006. Basic Steps in Planning Nursing Research: From Question to Proposal, sixth ed. Jones and Bartlett, Sudbury.

Surveys

Gathering data for research is exciting. However, its success depends largely on the method used. This must be appropriate to the research question, and should be a reasonable choice for the sample group. In this chapter we examine the use of the survey, which has traditionally been a popular method of collecting research information. A survey is defined as a method of gathering data by directly asking respondents for information in the form of either a questionnaire or an interview.

This chapter will examine some of the principles involved in the use of surveys, and examine the advantages and disadvantages of one method; the use of questionnaires. The principles of questionnaire design will be illustrated at the end of the chapter. The following chapter will examine the use of interviews.

THE SURVEY

The survey is a quantitative research design that collects written or verbal information from large numbers of individuals, through either the use of questionnaires or interviews, in an attempt to describe a situation in the form of numbers. It also provides a way of identifying correlation or patterns amongst some of the variables included in the survey. This allows the health researcher to have a better understanding of patterns of behaviour or reactions to the provision of health services that will help in the evidence-based planning and delivery of care. Houser (2008) claims the survey has become one of the most common method of data collection in nursing research, and midwifery researchers have also found this method of collecting data ideally suits many of the questions they wish to answer.

Why are surveys so popular? One reason is that they are very user friendly. They are less intimidating for both the researcher and those participating in comparison to some of the other forms of data collection. They are also a very economic way of collecting a large amount of data, illustrating the very practical reasons for their popularity. They are also an incredibly useful way of filling in gaps in our knowledge, as the number of results from surveys announced in the media every day testifies. Polit and Beck (2008: 324) illustrates this usefulness by saying:

> The greatest advantage of survey research is its flexibility and broadness of scope. It can be applied to many populations, it can focus on a wide range of topics, and its information can be used for many purposes.

In summary, surveys are widely accepted as a legitimate foundation for decision making in society. Their use has always been a feature of assessing maternity services, by both health professionals and consumer groups. This pattern is likely to increase in all areas of health care with the importance placed on user involvement under clinical governance.

The basic principle on which surveys are based is that if you want to know what is going on, then the best way to find out is to ask people. The results can include quantitative data in the form of numbers, or qualitative data in the form of words, with many surveys blending the two to give ideas about frequency backed up with comments on interpretations, experiences or opinions.

Surveys can vary in a number of ways, one of the most important being the degree of structure they contain. Very structured surveys are useful if the researcher wants to gain some idea of the kind of pattern involved with a certain type of activity, such as the number of women who intend to breastfeed, or the information needs of first-time pregnant mothers. This type of survey has the great advantage that the results are reasonably easy to analyse, as it usually involves counting the number who said 'yes' or 'no' or the numbers choosing each of the options in a list. This method is also a common method within audit, where a snapshot of a particular activity in one clinical area is produced.

However, the disadvantage of this method, as Polit and Beck (2008) observe, is that it can be superficial and still leave us asking 'why' in relation to a particular pattern of behaviour or opinion. More in-depth information can be gathered using a less structured data collection tool. However, with a less structured approach the researcher can be faced with information overload, and the answers may be very different from each other, making comparisons and summaries difficult.

A further variation is the time period examined by the survey. It can cover a 'one-off' collection of data, sometimes referred to as a *'cross-sectional survey'*, which considers the characteristics, experiences or views of those in a variety of clear subgroups in a population. The same survey can be repeated after a period of time with different groups to identify possible changes. For example, the number of women wanting a home birth could be gathered at one point, and then repeated one or more years later to see if there has been a change. This is known as a *trend survey*, and works in the same way as audit where the same measurement is used at different times on different people to gain an indication of changes.

A different form of the survey is the *longitudinal study*, which can follow the same group of people over time and keep going back to them to note any changes. This is sometimes called a *panel study* where the researcher returns to the same group of people over time to identify trends or changes (Burns and Grove 2009). One form of the longitudinal study is the *cohort study*, which follows one specific group of respondents over time (McKenna et al. 2010). This usually tracks the members of the group to establish possible influences of specific conditions. An example would be the study of a group of babies born to first-time mothers in one maternity unit in one month, who are followed-up over a 10-year period to plot any differences in childhood illnesses that might be influenced by type of infant feeding. The purpose of such studies is usually to identify risk factors for certain conditions (Houser 2008). A major problem with all types of studies that include repeated collections of survey data from the same group is people dropping out of the study (called 'study mortality'). Where this results in large numbers of people being lost to the study, it is likely to be difficult to develop any clear conclusions because of the amount of missing data.

There are two further problems concerning the use of surveys: the first relates to the representativeness of the sample, and the second relates to validity, or what is actually being measured. The issue relating to the sample is important, as the researcher frequently wishes to generalise the findings to similar people in the wider population. For this reason, researchers must try to avoid bias in the way the sample is chosen. Other methods of sampling will be covered in Chapter 14. Naturally, to get a reasonable picture of what is going on through the survey, the numbers returning questionnaires must be large and should as far as possible be representative of the total group. This is not always the case, which weakens the use of surveys in evidence-based practice, as it is often difficult to know if the results provide a true or accurate picture.

In designing the survey, it is usual to collect some basic 'demographic' details such as age, grade of staff, sex or number of children, so that some comparison can be made with those in the wider population to establish if they are a close comparison. This then gives some indication of how far the sample is representative.

The second question relating to validity is a difficult issue. One of the problems in surveys is that we have to accept that the answer given by a respondent is true, despite being unable to test it. There are likely to be some respondents who give socially acceptable answers in surveys, that is, answers that suggest the 'perfect citizen', so the accuracy can never be 100% certain. The only action the researcher can take is to try to reduce the amount of distortion produced by the data collection tool. The pilot study is one method by which this can be attempted.

THE USE OF QUESTIONNAIRES

Questionnaires are a tool of data collection consisting of a series of questions that are usually completed by the participants themselves (*self-completing*) and can take the form of paper, electronic text sent by email, or on-line versions. They collect information on such things as personal attributes, attitudes, beliefs experiences, behaviour and activities (Parahoo 2008), and are probably the most familiar data collection tool in nursing and midwifery research. Most of us are likely to have completed many questionnaires in our working lives, and perhaps deleted or thrown many more away. In this section we will examine some of the advantages and disadvantages of this method and outline some of the important principles of questionnaire design.

A large number of research questions in midwifery have been answered by questionnaire. Why are they such a popular method of collecting research data? Box 9.1 suggests some of the answers.

Although this list suggests that questionnaires are an ideal data collection method, several factors may discourage a response, as Box 9.2 suggests. There are, then, a balancing number of disadvantages to the use of questionnaires. However, people have now received so many questionnaires that their motivation to complete and return yet another may be low, resulting in a poor *response rate*, that is, the number of those retuning a questionnaire expressed as proportion of those receiving one. As Burns and Grove (2009) suggest, if the response rate is below 50%, the representativeness of the sample returned can be seriously in question, as there is no certainty that the responses represent the views of those sent a questionnaire. In other words, we may end up with a biased response. Generalisations from this group would then be impossible. Reminders can be sent to increase the final response rate, although the return from this may also be disappointingly low.

Similarly, a further limitation to their use is the often overlooked assumption that questionnaire recipients can read and write in English. This is not simply an issue of literacy or English not being a first language; many people have trouble with eyesight or problems with the ability to write because of physical problems. For this reason, surveys involving the public can omit important opinions because certain groups are excluded through the choice of research method.

The disadvantages of questionnaires relate to both the researcher and the respondent. A recurring frustration for the researcher is receiving returned questionnaires containing a number of unanswered questions, or incomplete

---

BOX 9.1 Advantages of questionnaires

Cheap
Quick
Can reach a large geographically spread sample
Can be quite detailed
Low level of embarrassment or threat to both researcher and respondent
Anonymity is protected
Fixed-choice questions easy to answer and to analyse
Familiar method to respondents

BOX 9.2 Disadvantages of questionnaires

Questionnaires have now saturated the population
Response rate may be low dependent on feelings on the topic
Questionnaires are dependent on reading levels, literacy skills and physical ability
Responses will be influenced by the quality of the design and the motivation used to produce a response
There is no opportunity for clarification of questions or answers
Fixed-choice questions may not have an appropriate option for everyone

answers. Once returned, it is not possible to clarify answers or probe further. From the respondent's point of view, one irritating feature of questionnaires is to be asked to choose from a range of options where none apply to their own situation. This raises questions of validity where a respondent is not truly describing his or her own views or experiences but merely choosing something the researcher has preselected. A final problem is where the researcher uses value-leaden words such as 'unnecessary', 'painful', 'appropriate', 'satisfied, 'too long', instead of phrasing questions in a neutral way. The conclusion is that as a method the questionnaire has a number of advantages and disadvantages. They are surprisingly not an easy option to use in research, and have a number of restrictions and limitations. Their success depends on the design, as this will influence whether an individual will complete them or not. For this reason, the next section will consider some of the principles involved in questionnaire design.

QUESTIONNAIRE DESIGN

The first stage in designing a questionnaire is to ensure that it is an appropriate method for collecting the data. Careful consideration should be given to the advantages and disadvantages outlined above. The study aim should also provide some clue as to whether it is appropriate. If the aim depends on finding out what people say or do, or relates to areas where individuals are in the best position to accurately supply the information, then questionnaires would seem a good option. The review of the literature should help to establish whether previous studies have used a questionnaire, and with what success. Once a final decision has been made to use a questionnaire then the researcher moves into the design stage. This does present a challenge, as Parahoo (2008: 300) observes:

> Developing questionnaires is systematic, time-consuming and laborious, requiring much preparation before the first question is phrased.

This can be made easier by following some clear principles. First, divide the questionnaire into its main parts:

- invitation and motivation to take part,
- instructions,
- body of the questionnaire.

INVITATION AND MOTIVATION TO TAKE PART

This section has traditionally been referred to as the 'covering letter' but with the variety of ways in which questionnaires are distributed, including web-based and emailed questionnaires it is better to talk about the invitations and motivation to take part (see Box 9.3). As Polit and Beck (2008) point out, this is the first contact potential respondents will have with the study, so it is important that it strikes the right balance that will prompt a reply. It should explain the purpose of the study and why they have been asked to take part. There should also be something that motivates the individual to give up time to participate. This might be by simply suggesting that it will help improve the service for others.

> **BOX 9.3** Elements that should be Included in an invitation
>
> Who you are and the capacity in which you are writing (e.g. student, member of a clinical team, or manager)
> The aim of the study, in broad terms
> The reason why the person has been included in the study
> Motivation to return the questionnaire (how they, or others, will benefit from completing it)
> Assurance on confidentiality and anonymity
> Estimate of the time is should take to complete
> Contact address/telephone number, should the respondent want further details or assurances
> Confirmation that the study has been given ethical approval

INSTRUCTIONS

The questionnaire should start with a clear title that summarises the purpose of the survey. The first section should be clearly marked 'Instructions'. This should simply and unambiguously outline the various ways questions can be answered, such as tick a box, click on an option or add a comment of their own. The pilot study should test the clarity of the instructions as, unless these are successful, valuable data may be lost.

THE MAIN BODY OF THE QUESTIONNAIRE

The 'business' part of the questionnaire is the body of questions. This section should look attractive and inviting, with good layout and space, as well as clean formatting of the questions and answers on the page. Cluttered and boring-looking questionnaires will not tempt people to answer them. Here we must ensure minimum margin for misunderstandings of the questions. The respondent should find it interesting and easy to complete, and the researcher should find that the replies provide an answer to the study aim. If this is to be achieved, then thought has to be given to:

- choice of questions,
- wording and structure of the questions,
- method of answering,
- analysis of the responses.

The choice of questions

The choice of the questions will be influenced by the research aim and the thinking that lies behind it. Where the researcher believes that a number of variables such as parity, previous experience and attitudes towards childbirth influence a situation, these should be included in the questions. The review of the literature will also provide some pointers to relevant questions.

At the design stage there is frequently a temptation to include too many questions. The longer the questionnaire, the less likely it is to be returned.

Every question should be relevant to the aim of the research. It is worth the researcher asking 'why am I including this question?'. If a clear answer cannot be given, the question should be deleted. It is also an advantage to ask colleagues, and particularly 'experts' in the field, for their view on the choice of topic areas and questions.

The wording and structure of the questions

The wording and structure of the questions need special attention. First, Box 9.4 outlines some of the basic principles of questionnaire design and, although these seem straightforward, they are frequently ignored. One piece of advice is to put yourself in the place of the person completing it; will it make sense to them? Are there certain assumptions being made about the person's knowledge that may not be justified? In following this advice it may be possible to avoid mistakes such as asking questions that are not

---

BOX 9.4 Basic principles in questionnaire design

Give clear instructions on how to answer the questions
Give assurances on confidentiality and only ask for name and identifying characteristics (e.g. clinical area if staff) if necessary
Questions should relate to the study aim
Avoid long questionnaires
Avoid long questions; respondents might lose track of its purpose
Avoid a single question asking more than one thing at the same time; split these into separate questions
Use simple language and avoid unnecessary or unexplained jargon and abbreviations
Use a clear layout to make it attractive on the page, and allow realistic space for written comments
Group questions on the same topic together to form a logical sequence
Avoid ambiguous questions and vague words such as 'regularly'
Avoid leading questions and value-loaded words
Avoid presuming that people do things; ask filter questions first
Avoid questions with 'no', 'not', 'never' in the question where the alternative answers are 'yes', or 'no' as it can lead to confusion
Ensure with fixed-choice questions that there is an alternative for everyone, such as 'not applicable', 'don't know' or 'other'
If people are unlikely to say 'yes' or 'no' to a question because of social desirability (looking good) then the question is not worth including
Use Likert scales ('strongly agree', etc. 'often', 'sometimes', 'rarely', 'never') where the answer may not be simply 'yes' or 'no'
Include a balance between open and closed questions to avoid repetitiveness
Leave sensitive, potentially embarrassing or intrusive questions until later in the questionnaire
At the design stage, think how you will analyse each question, even down to what a table of results will look like
Get comments on your draft questionnaire from colleagues and pilot it before using it to ensure it works (this should include analysis)

answerable. An example would be, 'Do you think the birth of your baby would have been better in a different hospital?' Not only does this give no indication as to what might count as 'better', it is clearly difficult for someone to evaluate whether there would have been differences if the birth had taken place in a different setting.

Vague words are a further problem in the wording of questions. There is a need for clarity of thought that should lead to precision in the wording of questions. Words such as 'regularly' should be avoided as in 'since the birth of your baby are you able to go out regularly'. This does not explain the context in which 'going out' is placed. Does it mean shopping, visiting people or social activities? Nor would it be meaningful as a 'yes' or 'no' response, as 'regularly' could mean vastly different things to different people.

As can be seen from the list of principles in Box 9.4, simplicity is one of the keys to questionnaire design. It is important to use simple words and to avoid jargon or technical terms such as 'primiparae' and 'multiparae' to non-medical people. Here, the reading level of the questionnaire needs careful assessment to ensure that people can understand each question (Houser 2008). The structure of each question should be simple and short and avoid asking more than one thing in a single sentence, such as:

Have you more than one child and were any of these born at home?
❏ YES ❏ NO

This should be divided into two; first it should ask 'have you more than one child' and then as a further sub-question: 'If 'yes', were any of these born at home?' This would then appear as follows:

5 a) *Have you more than one child?* ❏ YES ❏ NO
   b) *If yes, were any of these born at home?* ❏ YES ❏ NO

It is also important to avoid biasing the individual's response with leading questions or emotive words that suggest the appropriate answer, for example:

Would you agree that the midwife kept you fully informed during the labour?
Would it be more convenient for you to attend antenatal classes in a health centre near your home rather than in hospital?

This last question would be better asked in a more neutral way such as:

If you had a choice of where you could take part in antenatal education, which would you choose?
a) ❏ *Those at my local hospital*
b) ❏ *Those at my local health centre*
c) ❏ *Either one would be acceptable*
d) ❏ *Neither one would be acceptable*

The method of answering questions

The method of answering questions can take a number of forms. The final example above is called a multiple-choice question where the respondent chooses one of the alternatives offered. This falls into the category of *closed questions* as opposed to *open questions*. In open questions the respondent is not offered options to choose from, but is left to express the answer in his or her own words. An example of an open question would be the following:

What did you hope to gain from a home birth?

Open questions work well where respondents are used to expressing themselves in writing. They will not work well or be productive with everyone.

Open and closed questions have their advantages and disadvantages. For instance, although closed questions have the advantage of simplicity, they may influence the respondents by suggesting answers that they may not have thought of without the prompt of the fixed-choice options. The open question has the advantage of the respondent using terms and options that they feel describe their own experiences or views, rather than using those offered by the researcher. The disadvantage of open questions is the large amount of data that has to be analysed and coded before any kind of summary or identification of issues takes place. The ideal compromise is to have a mix of open and closed questions, which maximises the advantages of both forms of question.

One method of increasing the sensitivity of closed questions is the use of a range of scaling techniques (Burns and Grove 2009). Although we often think of closed questions as having a yes or no answer, where attitude or opinion is concerned, how people feel about an issue or statement may lie anywhere along a continuum. This can be dealt with using a *Likert scale*, which is named after the American, Rensis Likert, who first introduced them. These can take three forms and relate to:

- agreement,
- evaluation,
- frequency.

In the case of agreement scales, statements in a broad mix of positive or negative forms are given and the respondent is asked to make a choice between five choices ranging from 'strongly agree' to 'strongly disagree'. Fictional examples are shown below:

1. Agreement
   I feel that pain relief in labour should be taken as a last resort
   ❏ Strongly agree ❏ Agree ❏ Undecided
   ❏ Disagree ❏ Strongly disagree
2. Evaluation
   The information I received from the midwife about the alternative forms of pain relief was
   ❏ Excellent ❏ Very good ❏ Undecided
   ❏ Poor ❏ Very poor
3. Frequency
   I get feelings of panic when I think about looking after a baby
   ❏ Always ❏ Sometimes
   ❏ Rarely ❏ Never

In the last example, four choices have been used, as these seem to cover the main possibilities. The inclusion of 'never' removes the necessity to include a neutral midcategory. Some people argue that with examples 1. and 2. above, the midcategory of 'undecided' should be removed to prevent people choosing a neutral option and sitting on the fence (Houser 2008). From experience, this has never been seen in practice. It should also be remembered that there must be an option that applies to everyone. There are occasions when a midcategory could be a legitimate choice and should be respected.

The statements or 'items' in the Likert scale should be a mix of those expressed positively and those expressed negatively to prevent respondents simply putting a tick in the same column each time without really thinking about the question. So, for instance, the following two examples may be used in a satisfaction questionnaire.

The midwife was too busy to answer my questions
(negative item)
I felt confident with the midwife who conducted the birth
(positive item)

The order of these statements should not follow a set pattern, for instance, alternately positive and negative; providing there is an equal number of each kind of statement, they should be presented in a random order.

A similar technique to the Likert scale is to use a visual analogue scale (VAS) which is a line drawn across the page, usually 10 centimetres in length, with opposite words at each end. Respondents are asked to place a cross on the line to correspond with how they feel. This can either be calibrated with lines at centimetre points or can be assessed during the analysis by overlaying a calibrated piece of clear plastic on the line. This approach is often used in relation to pain. An example would be:

Mark with a cross on the line how you would describe your pain now
Worst pain imaginable   No pain at all

The analysis of the responses

The analysis of both the Likert scale and the visual analogue scale is treated in a similar way, by allocating a numeric value for the chosen response. In the case of the Likert scale a score of 5 is allocated for 'strongly agree' answers, 4 for 'agree', 3 for 'neither agree/disagree', 2 for 'disagree' and 1 for 'strongly disagree' when the statement is in the positive. When the statement is expressed in the negative, the reverse order of numbering would be applied (i.e. strongly disagree to the statement *'the midwife did not have time to answer my questions'* would be scored 5 to show there was a positive response to the midwife). An overall score for all the Likert questions can then be calculated for each person. It is also possible to give an average score for everyone in the sample. So, for instance, an average of 4.2 for the statement *'I felt confident with the midwife who helped me give birth'* would suggest that there was a high degree of satisfaction as the average was between the 'agree' and 'strongly agree' point on the scale. In the same way, the points on the visual analogue scale could be divided into 10 sections with each section given a score from 1 to 10, where 10 could be allocated to the positive end of the scale and 1 to the negative.

In questions requiring a 'yes' or 'no' answer, the responses can be expressed as a proportion of the total in terms of the percentage giving each response. The method of analysis should be carefully thought out at the design stage, and tested in the pilot and not left until the questionnaires start arriving back.

DETAILS OF HOW TO RETURN QUESTIONNAIRES

Although we have covered the three main parts of a questionnaire, we should also give thought to instructions on how to return the questionnaire to the researcher. If it has not been included in the instructions, the questionnaire should end with a 'thank you'. On-line questionnaires should indicate the end of the questionnaire has been reached and allow the respondent to 'submit', again with a 'thank you'. Paper questionnaires should clearly say how the questionnaire should be returned. This should be as simple as possible and should not involve the respondent in a complex or costly activity. It is this aspect that will influence the response rate and so should also be part of the pilot study to ensure it works smoothly.

ON-LINE SURVEYS

Finally, we consider the future of surveys and the use of on-line questionnaires, which are becoming increasingly popular. Although, this approach to data collection can be rich and valuable, Lagan (2010) observes very few midwifery researchers have explored this medium of conducting research.

As with all methodological issues, this approach has both advantages and disadvantages. Firstly, advantages would include the ease and speed of reply, both for the respondent and the researcher (Jones et al. 2008, Polit and Beck 2008). The number of people reached through such methods can be considerable and even world-wide (Lagan 2010). The method of analysis is easier as data does not have to be retyped but can be imported directly into a database for analysis and can give very fast results.

Clearly, there will be a number of disadvantages to the system, as it is still a new medium and lessons are still being learnt. However, early pioneers are already sharing their experiences and offering useful advice (Jones et al. 2008, Lagan 2010). As with postal questionnaires, there are concerns that the medium has inbuilt biases, such as the cross-section of potential respondents all need easy access to a computer, and essential computer skills. Respondents will still require reading, literacy and hand dexterity skills and this may form a barrier for some. Although postage costs are reduced compared to mailed questionnaires, there can be a design cost to such tools and technical knowledge skills related to Internet mediated research (IMR). However, this will continue to develop as a productive and growing area of midwifery research.

CONDUCTING RESEARCH

Although a survey provides quick and easy access to a large amount of data, the researcher should be cautious in the use of the questionnaire. This is because it is not always appropriate for those for whom writing is either not easy or not a welcome mental activity, or for those who have physical conditions, such as visual or handwriting problems. Even for those used to expressing themselves in writing, questionnaires have almost reached saturation point, and the motivation to complete and return a detailed questionnaire may be low.

Consideration must be given to the research aim, the sample, and the possible advantages of using another method, such as interviews. Ethical issues exist, and thought needs to be given to the possible harm through upset, anxiety or guilt caused by certain kinds of topic areas. These may include the loss of a baby, or the birth of a baby with a medical problem that may be thought to relate to maternal behaviour, such as smoking or dietary intake. Care should be taken, then, where the respondent may confront emotionally sensitive issues when they may be in a vulnerable mental state, and may have no one to help them through the distress caused by the questionnaire.

Where the decision to use the questionnaire is appropriate, it is important to avoid believing that designing appropriate questions is easy. The three elements, invitation to participate, instructions and main body of the questionnaire, need careful planning and design. The review of the literature will help identify appropriate topic areas, and may even give some pointers as to the kind of questions that have worked well in other studies. In selecting the wording of the questions, the researcher must keep validity and reliability in mind. The two important questions that need to be constantly addressed are:

- What am I trying to measure (validity)?
- How accurately will this question measure it (reliability)?

The basic principles of questionnaire design (see Box 9.4) should then be rigorously followed. Decisions on how the data resulting from each question are to be presented in a report/article should be considered at the question design stage. If you need statistical advice, it is at this stage at which it should be sought.

Questions should be as clear and as straightforward as possible. This means using simple language and simple sentences. Midwifery or medical jargon and abbreviations should be avoided as much as possible. It is not easy for the researcher to identify vague terms and ambiguity, as they have designed the question and are not confused by their meaning, so it is important to ask others to comment at the design stage.

Respondents should find a questionnaire interesting and enjoyable to complete. There should be variety in the way the questions are asked or required to be answered. The most frustrating experience for a respondent is to find that the choice of words clearly betrays the researcher's preconceived assumptions or personal agenda. This can be revealed through the use of emotive words such as 'better', 'disappointed', 'acceptable', and so on.

Using a questionnaire from a previous study is a big advantage; however, especially where a questionnaire has to be designed, a pilot study should be undertaken. In the pilot, it is important to have a good cross-section of the kinds of people who will be included in the main study. This is perhaps just as important as the size of the sample. The main questionnaire should be accompanied with a short questionnaire asking pilot respondents to identify any particular strengths or weaknesses in the main questionnaire. Relevant questions include:

- How long did it take you to complete the questionnaire?
- Were there any questions you had particular problems with?
- Was there any particular wording you had difficulty with?
- Are there any questions you feel were missing from the questionnaire?
- To sum up, what did you feel were the strengths of the questionnaire?
- What areas do you feel could be presented differently?

A 'practice' report based on the analysis of the data from the pilot should be produced to provide experience of moving from raw data to data presentation and analysis. At this point, serious shortcomings in the design of some questions, especially the method of answering, can be revealed.

CRITIQUING RESEARCH

Questionnaires are a popular method of data collection in midwifery; they have become so familiar that we rarely stop and challenge their use. We do need to ensure that the researcher has given a clear rationale for selecting a questionnaire rather than the usually more effective method of interviewing. Where the sample is geographically spread, or where an existing relationship between the researcher and participants may compromise the use of interviews, then questionnaires are an appropriate choice. It is worth considering any ethical issues raised by the use of the questionnaires with the topic, and whether the researcher has addressed these. For instance, we would be unhappy where a questionnaire was used to explore feelings about the loss of a baby, or similar subjects that may result in upset, anxiety or needlessly raising feelings of guilt, confusion or regret.

The space provided in some journals does not permit the inclusion of an entire questionnaire, so we should not expect the opportunity to judge each question. Sometimes, tables provide a clue as to the content and wording of the questionnaire. Where possible, place yourself in the position of the respondents and ask was there any possibility of ambiguity or misunderstanding? Are the questions in any way leading, for instance, the use of emotive words that suggests how the researcher felt about the topic?

What evidence is there that the researcher addressed the issue of reliability of the questions, especially if they were designed for the study and had not been used in previous studies? Was the accuracy of the questions tested through a pilot study? In regard to validity, how do we know the questions were measuring what they were supposed to measure? Did the researcher develop some of the questions from previous research, or were experts in the field approached to comment on the appropriateness of the topics for the study?

Finally, we should consider the researcher's interpretation of the results. Are the results strong enough to support the statements made by the researcher? We should also be aware that what people say they do may not be what they do in practice. In other words, we should always be somewhat cautious in treating self-reported data as if it were 'the truth'.

KEY POINTS

- Questionnaires enable a large amount of data to be collected quickly and cheaply. They have the advantage of being familiar to a majority of the population, and compared to other forms of data collection, are a non-threatening medium for both the researcher and respondent.
- The response rate is variable. Where it falls under 50%, it is difficult to be certain that the responses received are representative of the sample as a whole.
- Questionnaires have been used so often in the past that people are now less likely to return them. Is this the most appropriate method here? In particular, the ethical issue of harm should be considered where the questions could produce emotional upset, regret, anxiety or confusion.
- Designing a questionnaire involves three elements: the invitation, the instructions, and the body of the questionnaire. There are clear guidelines that should be followed in the construction of questions. The importance of avoiding bias and ensuring reliability and validity must be stressed.
- The basic premise of questionnaire design is that the respondent can read and write, and is fluent in the English language. For several reasons, there is a proportion of the population who will always be excluded in studies using questionnaires. Similarly, with electronic versions, not everyone has access to a computer.
- A pilot study, or the use of a previously used questionnaire, is a good indicator of rigour in the use of questionnaires.

REFERENCES

Burns, N., Grove, S., 2009. The Practice of Nursing Research: Appraisal, Synthesis, and Generation of Evidence. sixth ed. Saunders, St Louis.

Houser, J., 2008. Nursing Research: Reading, Using and Creating Evidence. Jones and Bartlett, Sudbury.

Jones, S., Murphy, F., Edwards, H., James, J., 2008. Doing things differently: advantages and disadvantages of web questionnaires. Nurse Res. 15 (4), 15–26.

Lagan, B., 2010. Internet-mediated research: a reflection on challenges encountered and lessons learnt. Evidence Based Midwifery 8 (1), 26–30.

McKenna, H., Hasson, F., Keeney, S., 2010. Surveys. In: Gerrish, K., Lacey, A. (Eds.), The Research Process in Nursing. sixth ed. Wiley-Blackwell, Chichester.

Parahoo, K., 2008. Questionnaires. In: Watson, R., McKenna, H., Cowman, S., Keady, J. (Eds.), Nursing Research: Designs and Methods. Churchill Livingstone, Edinburgh.

Polit, D., Beck, C., 2008. Nursing Research: Generating and Assessing Evidence for Nursing Practice. eighth ed. Lippincott Williams and Wilkins, Philadelphia.

Interviews

10

The last chapter considered one of the two main methods of collecting survey data: the questionnaire. Although popular with researchers, this is not always the most appropriate choice for a number of reasons, such as the poor response rate. Certainly for the mothers of new babies, sitting down to complete a questionnaire may be difficult to fit into a hectic lifestyle. Questionnaires have also become an overused medium for collecting research data.

Interviews are the second method of collecting data in surveys. These are used in a variety of research designs including qualitative research. Interviews have a great deal to offer midwifery research as the type of data produced tends to be richer and has more depth than is generally possible with questionnaires. Interviews also make use of the midwife's professional skill of sensitively, collecting information through a conversational medium. It can also increase the variation in the range of people included in a study.

In this chapter we examine some of the features of interviews, especially their advantages and disadvantages, and consider some of the skills involved in interviewing.

DEFINITION

Interviews consist of data gathering through direct interaction between a researcher and respondent where answers to questions are gathered verbally. They can take the form of face-to-face encounters, the telephone or the web. Although usually conducted on a one-to-one basis, they can be carried out with a group of individuals in the form of a *focus group*. These are small groups of individuals who are facilitated by the researcher to discuss certain topics and experiences.

Interviews are one form of data collection that is used in both quantitative and qualitative studies, and have the ability to describe, explain and explore issues from the individual or 'insider' perspective (Tod 2010). The research approach will influence the type of data collected and method of data analysis. One important advantage of interviews over other methods of data collection is the higher response rate than with other methods (Burns and Grove 2009). In qualitative research, they have become the most common type of method of

© 2011 Elsevier Ltd. All rights reserved.

data collection (Holloway and Wheeler 2010). However, from the researcher's perspective, they present some of the greatest challengers and the need for a high level of skills in their use. To a large extent, the researcher *becomes* the tool of data collection in studies using this method. This is because, although interviews may be recorded in writing on a printed form or in a notebook, or verbally on audio equipment and later transcribed, it is the researcher's skills and personality that will encourage or discourage the interviewee to open up and select the information they feel willing to disclose. During interviews, it is also the researcher's ability to know when to seek clarification or illustration that can make all the difference to the quality of the data collected.

INTERVIEW STRUCTURE

Interviews can be categorised by the degree of structure they contain. This can range from a highly structured format of questioning, where they virtually take the form of reading out questions from a questionnaire and recording the answers. This approach is used in survey designs that concentrate on the production of quantitative data. Here, the list of questions is not called a questionnaire but an *interview schedule* (Jackson et al. 2008). The advantages of this format, according to Bryman (2008), include the standardisation in the way questions are asked and recorded. This increases the accuracy of the results and also makes analysis easier and more compatible with statistical computer analysis programmes. The disadvantage of a highly structured approach is that there is little scope for spontaneity and depth of information. This can result in them being somewhat superficial, leaving us with little understanding of a situation. We must also remember that, as a self-report method, we have to assume that what someone states in an interview is accurate.

At the other end of the interview structure continuum is the *unstructured or non-standardised interview* where questions develop as appropriate with a participant. This allows situations to be seen through the eyes of those involved, a point made by Polit and Beck (2008: 392):

> Unstructured interviews encourage respondents to define the important dimensions of a phenomenon and to elaborate on what is relevant to them rather than being guided by the investigator's a priori notions of relevance.

This means that rather than choose from what the researcher has decided are relevant options, the respondent can put what they see as important in their own words, so we get an insider's description of events and issues. Such interviews have only a small number of prepared questions, called an *interview guide*; the rest will be requests for more detail or illustration. Often, they may start with a trigger question or *grand tour question* (Polit and Beck 2008), such as, 'So what happened once you went into labour?' The disadvantage of the approach is that it requires a great deal of personal skill from the researcher and generates a large amount of data to be analysed and coded, and so can be very time consuming and costly.

Somewhere between these two extremes are *semi-structured interviews*, which are a mixture of the two. They contain some standard questions covering issues or topic areas that are asked of everyone (Holloway and Wheeler 2010), but there is also the flexibility to probe and explore areas that seem appropriate to the individual concerned. The semi-structured approach ensures that important areas are covered with everyone, but still allows other areas to arise spontaneously.

ADVANTAGES AND DISADVANTAGES OF INTERVIEWS

Why choose interviews as a data collection method? There are a number of very clear advantages to using interviews, as can be seen from Box 10.1. According to Polit and Beck (2008: 424), these strengths far outweigh those of questionnaires. They are suitable for a wider variety of individuals than questionnaires, are less likely to lead to misinterpretations of the questions, and provide richer data. The presence of the interviewer can also be an asset as they can clarify questions and answers and gently probe where more information may be needed to gain a complete and accurate answer. This has been recognised by Burns and Grove (2009: 405), who suggest that interviews allow the researcher to explore a greater depth of meaning than can be obtained with other methods.

Interviews have a particular relevance in midwifery as they provide an opportunity to pursue a woman-centred approach to issues and situations. This is particularly the case in semi-structured and unstructured interviews, as their purpose is to hear 'the voice' of the participants, so as to enable an understanding of the situation from their perspective (Holloway and Wheeler 2010).

As with all the other methods of data collection presented in this book, we have to be aware of their disadvantages. The main issues are outlined in Box 10.2. One of the main issues is that successful interviews not only depend on the high skill levels of the interviewer, but also depend on the interviewee being articulate and reflective on their experiences or thoughts (Jackson et al. 2008). A number of other issues relate to the practicalities of the technique. They require a great deal of time per interview in terms of both gathering the data and their analysis, particularly where the interview is semi-structured or unstructured. This naturally increases the cost of such research.

A further problem is the influence of the interviewer on the information produced. The fact that this is a social situation means that the characteristics of each of the individuals concerned can play a part in the reliability and

---

BOX 10.1 Advantages of interviews

Suitable for a wide range of people including those who have a problem with literacy, visual problems, and are suitable for mothers and health professionals who have little time to complete questionnaires
Response rate is usually higher than with questionnaires
Presence of an interviewer reduces misunderstandings and the number of missed questions
Participants can feel more in control in semi-structured and unstructured interviews and therefore feel more valued
In-depth responses can be gained, allowing the participants 'voice' to emerge
Information is immediately available for analysis
Overall better quality data in comparison to questionnaires

> **BOX 10.2 Disadvantages of interviews**
>
> Interviewing is a highly skilled activity that requires careful training and practice
> Time consuming and costly to carry out and analyse in comparison to questionnaires
> Danger of participants providing 'socially acceptable' answers
> Participants can be influenced by the interviewer's status, characteristics or behaviour
> Participants can feel put on the spot, 'tested', or worry they will 'look a fool' if they answer completely honestly and so suffer from 'stage-fright' – as can the interviewer
> Some participants may not be used to expressing deep feelings or emotions openly to others or on reflecting on events or feelings

validity of the information produced. There is inevitably a conscious or subconscious influence on the selection and editing of information by the participant. Where the interviewer is a midwife or other health professional, no matter how much they encourage participants to see them as just someone interested in their experiences, there is a hierarchical position of the interviewer over the interviewee that may influence the outcome of some interviews. For example, *'socially desirable'* answers (those that put the person in a positive light) may be selected to impress or avoid possible criticism or rebuke from health staff. One final problem is where the participants 'second guesses' the answers on the basis of what they think the interviewer wants to hear. All these elements will have a negative effect on the validity of interview data.

PRINCIPLES IN THE USE OF INTERVIEW

Interviewing is a skill frequently practiced outside the gaze of those who need to learn from those who do it well. Although asking questions and receiving answers sounds deceptively easy as a method of data collection, like everything else in research, things are never that simple. However, it is possible to overcome some of the difficulties through knowledge of the pitfalls and by following some essential principles.

A major step is to recognize that research interviews are not like ordinary conversations, as their purpose is to elicit research data. Burns and Grove (2009: 404) warn that nurses and midwives may feel that because they frequently use the interview in clinical assessments, the dynamics of the interview are familiar; however, they emphasise that using the technique in research requires a greater sophistication. They go on to provide the following essential advice:

> *Skilled interviewing requires practice, and interviewers must be familiar with the content of the interview. They must anticipate situations that might occur during the interview and develop strategies for dealing with them.*

Their advice is for the interviewer to use role-play to develop appropriate skills and coping mechanisms. This firstly should be with colleagues, where it can be used very much like a rehearsal. These could be audio recorded or even visually recorded for playback later to identify appropriate skills and areas that need developing. This should, of course, be followed up later with a pre-test study with members from the group in whom the researcher is interested.

A major consideration in carrying out an interview is the location and characteristics of the environment in which the interview takes place. The participant should feel relaxed and comfortable. There should be as few disturbances and distractions as possible whilst the interview takes place. Although many people provide the best information in their own home, the interviewer's control over the setting is drastically reduced. Despite interruptions having an impact on the flow of information, sometimes this has to be accepted and may be inevitable, especially with a young baby around. One student told me of an interview she had undertaken in a respondent's home where there was not only a fierce-looking dog present, but also a rabbit running around. The woman being interviewed jumped up at one point to shoo away the rabbit after it had urinated on the dog's bedding for the third time, while the dog sat in a corner vomiting. All of this was captured on the audio recorder. Under these circumstances it is important the interviewer does not show any irritation, exasperation, surprise or disgust.

Interviews in a participant's home also raise issues of personal safety, and it is wise for researchers to ensure that people know where they are, and the timetable they are following. Researchers should also protect themselves by carrying such items as a mobile phone and alarm to enhance personal safety. Wherever the interview takes place, simple things such as ensuring that the sun is not shining in the participant's eyes and that they are comfortable are important, as this will affect the quality of the information produced.

The interviewer's appearance also needs careful thought so as to reduce producing socially desirable answers. The way the interviewer is dressed or the accessories worn could act as distractions, or indications of possible personal beliefs and values. Where possible, the interviewer's appearance should be relatively nondescript. In terms of etiquette, it is also important that the interviewer states the approximate length of time the interview may take and ensures that respondents are not worried about other responsibilities or obligations that may distract them as the interview lengthens.

The nature of the interview will also be influenced by the method of recording the answers. The two options are making written notes as the interview unfolds, or using an audio recorder (although visual recording is also possible, these are very rare). New technologies with video links through a computer may develop this further in the future. In relation to writing or audio recording of data, both have their advantages and disadvantages. Written notes are not as intimidating as using an audio recorder and the interviewer does not have to worry about background noise affecting the recording. There is also little risk of technology letting the researcher down, although it is important to have a good supply of pens or pencils that are in good working order! The disadvantage of writing is the inability to maintain eye contact with participants. This can be difficult for both interviewer and participant. It can feel somewhat like making a police statement rather than an interview. There is also an inevitable loss of information as it is rarely possible to write down everything that is said. The main difficulty for the researcher is coping with a racing mind that is thinking of the next question, remembering what has just been said, trying to remember how to spell tricky words and making a mental note of interesting comments that have just been made that will need to be probed or followed up later.

Audio recorders have the advantage of leaving the interviewer free to concentrate on the conversation rather than trying to speed-write everything. The ability to maintain eye contact can also be very important in interviews on sensitive topics. Apart from the problem of background noise, audio recorders are successful in capturing almost all of the comments from the participant in their own words. This can be a crucial advantage, particularly in qualitative research. The disadvantages of audio recorders include the fact that some participants find them intimidating. They are an additional worry for the interviewer, in case something goes wrong with them, such as batteries running out or recordings being lost. Almost every researcher has their 'bad experience' story of 'lost' interviews. Transcribing interviews can also take a very long time to complete.

TELEPHONE INTERVIEWS

Although interviews have traditionally been face to face, research methods have been quick to take advantage of new developments and technologies. One example is the use of telephone interviews. This section will briefly consider their advantages and disadvantages so that they can be used for their strengths.

Most authors are positive about the role of telephone interviews, providing they follow certain principles. For example, Polit and Beck (2008: 324) suggests:

> *Telephoning can be a convenient method of collecting information if the interview is short, specific, and not too personal, or if researchers have had prior personal contact with respondents.*

They work well in a quantitative design, as illustrated in the research by Scott et al. (2008). Their aim was to identify the incidence of mastitis in the first 6 months postpartum in a Scottish population of mothers. Breastfeeding women were recruited to the study prior to discharge home after completing a baseline questionnaire. They were then telephoned regularly to identify any symptoms of mastitis. If these were identified, they were asked to provide further information on the symptoms, the management and advice they received from health professionals. This is a far superior method in this study compared to either repeated face-to-face interviews or questionnaires.

Similarly, a study by Forster and McLachlan (2010) on women's views on breastfeeding 6 months postpartum used two open questions at the end of a telephone interview of approximately 60 questions to 889 mothers. They were asked: 'Overall, how do you feel about breastfeeding?' and 'Do you have any other comments on breast feeding (positive or negative)?' The replies were written down verbatim but no elaboration was requested.

Both these studies show a good use of the telephone interview and illustrate many of the advantages of the method. For example, Holloway and Wheeler (2010) emphasise their convenience for health professionals and health care recipients with little time for interviews, and they also save travel time for the researcher. In addition, they have an immediacy of response, anonymity for participants, and also make good use of project time. This is naturally helped by a highly structured format to the questions.

These advantages should be weighed against the potential disadvantages. Bryman (2008: 198) highlights a number of considerations, for instance the length of a call should not extend much more than 20 minutes, and he suggests they are not a good medium for pursing sensitive issues. The lack of visual cues also means that the researcher can be unaware of misunderstanding or confusion. Holloway and Wheeler (2010) also point out that they have the disadvantage of the limited depth of interaction because of these factors; Bryman (2008) agrees and adds that individuals tend to be less engaged with the interview process, and that this can result in a lower quality of data compared to the face-to-face interview.

The conclusion is that, as with other tools of data collection, the choice of telephone interview has to be matched with the research question, the sample, the type and extent of data required and comparisons made with the advantages of other forms of data collection.

FOCUS GROUPS

A further variation on the use of interview is the *focus group*, which has increasingly been used in health service research. Although thought to be quite modern and developed by market researchers, focus groups do have a long history in social research of over 80 years, when they were first used with soldiers in the Second World War (Redmond and Curtis 2009).

Focus groups are used where the concern is not so much on individual experiences and interpretations, but on how people who share things in common, such as pregnancy or recent birth, talk about the topic and share their experiences or views. They are also used where the purpose is to stimulate discussion and debate on a topic or issue (Goodwin and Happell 2009) or as a means of exploring a topic where little is known (Redmond and Curtis 2009). Their use is based on the premise that group settings can help people to express and clarify their views in ways that may not emerge in individual interviews. As with other qualitative approaches, the intension is to produce rich details on complex experiences.

The size of such groups does vary but most authors suggest numbers in the region of four to eight. The researcher running such groups is called a *moderator*, and sometimes a second researcher taking notes and observes the interactions between participants.

There are disadvantages. For example Joyce (2008) suggests that the individual interview still has clear advantages over the focus group when it comes to the level of control and the amount of information gathered from each participant. This is supported by Burns and Grove (2009), who cite the conclusion of market researchers that in-depth interviews provide better value and quality data than focus groups. A great deal of their success is based on the skills of the moderator, who has to ensure that all individuals are encouraged to participate and that the topic is explored in depth. This demonstrates that this method should not be used simply as a cheap way of collecting information.

One midwifery example is the work of Pitchforth et al. (2009) where the aim was to explore women's perceptions and experiences of 'choice' of place of birth in remote and rural areas in the north of Scotland. The study consisted of 12 focus groups, each with an average of six participants, although numbers varied from four to nine members. A semi-structured interview guide was used, where women were asked to consider: the choices they were given about place of birth, which factors they considered when making their decision, and who or what had influenced the decision-making process. Within the discussion, the groups were presented with one scenario-based question which asked them to choose between a consultant-led unit, a midwife managed unit and a home birth. Each group's discussions lasted between 45 minutes and one hour. The findings are presented as themes that emerged from the discussions. The women felt they were not offered a real choice as to where they had their baby, and any options were restricted, with the final decision frequently made for them. When faced with the scenario of the different models of care, decisions were influences by issues of safety and the social and personal financial implications of the various choices. Often, this related to travelling time and costs for relatives to visit them immediately following the birth. In this study, focus groups were an appropriate choice of method, as the aim was to identify different experiences in where women gave birth, and to identify the influences on the views of these women on appropriate places to give birth. The focus groups also enabled the researches to access these women in rural communities by bringing together volunteers from those already attending mother and toddler groups in the local areas.

INTERVIEWING SKILLS

The success of this type of research is greatly influenced by the interviewing skills of the researchers. Clearly, a skilled interviewer will produce higher-quality data than one with poorer skills (Burns and Grove 2009). What makes a good interview? Good interviews are the result of more than asking the questions clearly, although that does help. One key is to establish rapport with respondents (Jackson et al. 2008), which can be defined as an understanding and close relationship between people. This means producing a friendly atmosphere where individuals feel respected and comfortable with the researcher enough to trust them with sensitive information without fear of judgement, criticism or ridicule. Non-verbal skills are also required, including the seating position of the interviewer in relation to the participant; if they are square-on, almost in a head-to-head position, the participant may feel it is more like an interrogation rather than a relaxed conversation. Sitting slightly to the side of the individual, where eye contact can be made, helps to establish the right atmosphere. It is important that this is at a comfortable distance from the individual, so that they do not feel that their personal space is being restricted or invaded.

Comfortable eye contact is also part of non-verbal skills, and the researcher leaning slightly forward to indicate that they are listening also encourages rapport. Interviewers should avoid crossing their arms or legs, as this might suggest they are nervous, or keeping information secret from the respondent.

The key principle is to relax; if the interviewer is relaxed, it will encourage the respondent to relax also.

It is also important to consider the process of closing the interview. The researcher should thank the respondents and ask them if there are any things they feel have not been covered or said so far. The researcher should offer the participant the opportunity to ask any questions of the interviewer. This allows any concerns or important questions that may have come to the participant's mind during the course of the interview to be identified. This is a clear demonstration of the kind of the reciprocity or balance of 'give and take' that should exist in interviews, where the researcher should share any expertise or knowledge with the participant.

The skills of interviewing with focus groups are somewhat different, as the setting and issues that arise are not the same as with individual interviews because of the group context. For instance, one problem is the possible domination of the group by one or more very vocal or strong characters (Goodwin and Happell 2009). A further problem identified by Goodwin and Happell (2009) is how to keep track of who has said what, especially where groups are audio recorded. The authors suggest a tracking sheet to identify individual responses so that variations in experiences and views can be attributed to those within the group without confusing who said what. However, where there are rapid exchanges of conversation, keeping track of who is speaking and marking this on a sheet can be very difficult.

CONDUCTING RESEARCH

Interviews should be considered when the research question suggests a self-report method appropriate to a face-to-face setting, either one-to-one or focus group. Focus groups are useful for establishing how a specific group talks about and experiences issues in which the researcher is interested. Although interviewing a group may seem a cheaper method than interviewing the same number individually, they are used for different reasons and will not always achieve the same outcomes.

Both alternatives are useful where the individual may not have considered the subject in any depth or may not feel his or her views are important enough to return a questionnaire. Similarly, they should be considered where the topic might need to be explored with the help of the researcher, or one that may produce some depth that could not be captured by a questionnaire. Interviews are a good choice where the aim of the study is to explore a topic through the eyes of the participant and the researcher wants participants to recount their experiences in some depth in their own words.

One special situation requiring a lot of thought is interviews conducted with health professionals, particularly where those to be interviewed know or are known by the interviewer. This is a very different situation from interviewing strangers, as past histories can interfere with the quality of data produced and where the social distance needed to explore certain topics with strangers does not exist (Burns and Grove 2009). However, Burns and Grove (2009) also point out that insider knowledge can be useful, particularly in the interpretation of the results or in picking up subtleties that might be missed by a researcher unfamiliar with the setting.

Once the interview has been chosen as the appropriate tool, the researcher must consider the degree of structure it will contain, ranging from structured through to semi-structured and unstructured. The more unstructured options are often chosen were little is known about the topic (Tod 2010). Whichever degree of structure, researchers must ensure they are fully trained and experienced in undertaking the role of interviewer. Rehearse with colleagues using an audio recorder, and listen to your strengths and areas for improvement. Be relaxed and establish 'rapport' so respondents feel you are friendly, non-judgmental and that they can trust you. However, you have a job to do. Although you are listening and valuing what the person is saying, you are not doing so passively, and you must analyse 'on air' the contribution this is making to the research question. For example, should you consider asking for more detail, or change the topic? In this way, you are the tool of data collection and this requires tremendous skill, focus and awareness of the simultaneous task you are undertaking if the person's time is going to be fully respected.

The body language of the interviewer is fundamental in helping the participant to relax in potentially stressful and intimidating situation. There are many skills involved in the interview, for example, active listening and avoiding rephrasing the participant's answer in one's own words, as this can lead to bias. In addition, where it is clear that the participant has decided to describe a particular topic or account rather than an alternative, the interviewer must consider whether to bring them back to that point later and explore the alternative. Where an interruption or deviation in conversation occurs, the interviewer may have to help the respondent to return to the place reached before the interruption or change in direction.

Anything can happen in a free-flowing interview. An important warning is that while telling their 'story', respondents can relive painful memories, and experience heightened emotional responses. If a memory is stressful or painful, the respondent may exhibit anger, fear, sadness or distress. Under these circumstances a decision has to be made on whether the interview should be abandoned or delayed until the participant recovers. However, some people find these emotional moments therapeutic. Individuals can sometimes feel grateful for the opportunity to have someone at last listen and acknowledge their experiences and feelings.

Where an interview is particularly intense, it is possible for the feelings of closeness with the interviewer to lead to the participant revealing 'secrets'. It should be remembered that where the interviewer is a midwife, the professional code of conduct does not allow all information to be kept secret (see Chapter 8 on ethics). Examples would be anything related to a child or mother, abuse or neglect, or a report of poor or unacceptable professional conduct. Under these circumstances the midwife cannot continue in the researcher role of keeping the information confidential but has a duty to report it. If the situation arises where a participant indicates that they want to share something that they declare is confidential, the midwife interviewer must stop them and make the researcher's own position clear before the participant says something that might be regretted later.

These points emphasise the exhausting nature of interviews, especially those relating to very sensitive areas. It is possible for the researcher to absorb a great deal of other people's emotions that must then be dealt with. For this reason, avoid conducting more than a small number of interviews per day and have a good research supervisor or mentor who can help deal in a positive way with the emotional after-effects of interviewing. Finally, interviews may involve entering into someone's emotional life, so, as Tod (2010) warns, the decision to use this method should not be taken without careful consideration. The researcher can feel a sense of betrayal and exploitation in sharing data or experiences where they have arisen in very poignant and private circumstances. Despite these words of warning, interviews can be exhilarating, richly rewarding and provide real insights into key areas of life that cannot easily be gained using other methods.

CRITIQUING RESEARCH

In critiquing a research article based on interviews, the first question to ask is, 'was it an appropriate choice of data collection tool?'. In other words, would the disadvantages of the interview have suggested that an alternative method might have been more appropriate? We also need some indication of the degree of structure in the interview that may have encouraged or curtailed the views of the respondent, and the language in which they could respond; the more the interview was structured, the less it is possible to express views in the participant's own words.

One problem with many research reports is that it is difficult to get an idea of the conditions under which the interview took place. We frequently have no idea of the possible strength and weakness that may have influenced the reliability of the interview. In most instances, although the person undertaking the interview might be named, we have little idea of their appearance at the time of the interviews, and how they were dressed. Where the interviewer was a midwife, did the participants know them, and were they in uniform? Both these factors might influence the findings.

We should look for some assurance that the researcher followed principles to increase the quality of the data; for instance, did he or she practice the interview with either colleagues or with those from the study group, and did he or she return some interviews back to those involved for verification? The method of analysis of the findings should also be described and be credible, for example, naming a type of data analysis or the name of someone whose method of analysis has been applied to the data.

The presentation of results should also be examined. Although selection and editing is inevitable, it is still important that themes and key examples of issues are relevant to the aim of the study and based on a cross-section of those contributing to the study.

Finally, remember, as with questionnaires, that interviews are self-report methods and rely on the accuracy of what people say and the extent to which this truly reflects actions and beliefs. For this reason, there is always a limit to generalisations made from interview data.

KEY POINTS

- Interviews have many advantages over questionnaires. In midwifery, they also have the advantage of being compatible with a woman-centred approach to care. They can be used to collect quantitative data using a structured interview schedule, or qualitative data using a semi-structured, or unstructured format.
- Semi-structured and unstructured interviews have the advantage of collecting rich data through the interactive form of the interview. They provide a unique view of events as seen by those receiving services or those experiencing parenthood. The results are frequently unexpected, illuminating, and can differ from the perspective of health professionals.
- There are a number of disadvantages to interviews. They are costly and time consuming. The physical presence of the researcher can also be intimidating to some participants, and the resulting data can be consciously or subconsciously skewed in the direction of socially desirable answers. They also require a high level of skill on the part of the interviewer to avoid some of the pitfalls outlined.
- The time-consuming nature of interviews means that sample size is frequently smaller than that possible with questionnaires. However, this does not automatically limit their usefulness, especially within qualitative research.

REFERENCES

Bryman, A., 2008. Social Research Methods, third ed. Oxford University Press, Oxford.

Burns, N., Grove, S., 2009. The Practice of Nursing Research: Appraisal, Synthesis, and Generation of Evidence. sixth ed. Saunders, St Louis.

Forster, D., McLachlan, H., 2010. Women's views and experiences of breast feeding: positive, negative or just good for the baby? Midwifery 26 (1), 116–125.

Goodwin, V., Happell, B., 2009. Seeing both the forest and the trees: a process for tracking individual responses in focus group interviews. Nurse Res. 17 (1), 62–67.

Holloway, I., Wheeler, S., 2010. Qualitative Research for Nurses. third ed. Wiley-Blackwell, Chichester.

Jackson, D., Daly, J., Davidson, P., 2008. Interviews. In: Watson, R., McKenna, H., Cowman, S., Keady, J. (Eds.), Nursing Research: Designs and Methods. Churchill Livingstone, Edinburgh.

Joyce, P., 2008. Focus groups. In: Watson, R., McKenna, H., Cowman, S., Keady, J. (Eds.), Nursing Research: Designs and Methods. Churchill Livingstone, Edinburgh.

Pitchforth, E., van Teijlingen, E., Watson, V., et al., 2009. 'Choice' and place of delivery: a qualitative study of women in remote and rural Scotland. Qual. Saf. Health Care 18, 42–48. doi: 10.1136/qshc.2007.023572.

Polit, D., Beck, C., 2008. Nursing Research: Generating and Assessing Evidence for Nursing Practice. eighth ed. Lippincott Williams and Wilkins, Philadelphia.

Redmond, R., Curtis, E., 2009. Focus groups: principles and process. Nurse Res. 16 (3), 57–69.

Scott, J., Robertson, M., Fitzpatrick, J., Knight, C., Mulholland, S., 2008. Occurrence of lactational mastitis and medical management: A prospective cohort study in Glasgow. International Breastfeeding Journal 3 (21). doi: 10.1186/1746-4358-3-21.

Tod, A., 2010. Interviewing. In: Gerrish, K., Lacey, A. (Eds.), The Research Process in Nursing. sixth ed.. Wiley-Blackwell, Chichester.

Observation

In the last two chapters, questionnaires and interviews have been described as methods that gather data on what people do and think by asking them directly. One of the major difficulties of these two methods is that we have to assume that what people say they do is accurate. Observation differs in that it collects information first hand, based on what people are seen to do by the researcher.

The aim of this chapter is to consider the reasons for using observation as a method, and to identify some of its advantages and disadvantages. Two approaches to observation will be highlighted. Firstly, the quantitative method of checklist observation will be briefly mentioned, and secondly, qualitative approaches to observation will be outlined in more detail. Although observation is used less frequently than questionnaires and interviews, there are a number of classic observational studies in midwifery, and one of these will be mentioned later.

WHAT IS OBSERVATION?

We are observing the world around us all the time, so what is the difference between 'looking' and 'observing' in research terms? The answer, according to Wood and Ross-Kerr (2006: 171), is that observation stops being part of normal human activity and becomes a research method when it is systematically planned and recorded and when the results are checked for their accuracy. In other words, observation is different from looking when it is carried out systematically for the purpose of answering a research question to develop knowledge. Observation can be defined as the collection of data that are visible to visual sensors, whether that consists of the researcher's eyes or the use of some means of visual recording. Watson et al. (2010: 382) add that as a tool of data collection, 'observation is an active process by which data are collected about people, behaviours, interactions or events'.

As with interviews (Chapter 10), observation varies depending on the amount of structure used to record the data. At one extreme is the highly *structured observation* checklist that produces quantitative data and at the other is the *unstructured observation* of situations that are used to produce qualitative data.

© 2011 Elsevier Ltd. All rights reserved.

In the last chapter, researchers were seen as the tool of data collection in the way they channelled the verbal information in the form of an interview. In this chapter, researchers are again the tool of data collection in the way in which they select and record the data they 'see' to answer the research aim. Indeed, Mcilfatrick (2008: 310) suggests that observation 'epitomises the idea of the researcher as the research instrument'.

WHY USE OBSERVATION?

We have repeatedly noted that although we can ask people what they do, we may not always get an accurate answer. This is because people are not always aware of what they do, or they are unable to accurately describe or articulate their actions. Some actions are carried out at a subconscious level and are difficult to describe or write down. Explaining how to tie a shoelace to someone over the phone is a good example. Data gathering using observation can overcome the problem of verbal descriptions. It can be applied to numerous midwifery activities where the best way to find out how someone does something or 'what happens' in certain situations is to watch it unfold. One example of this is the work by Kemp and Sandall (2010) who observed five 36-week birth talks in women's homes by their caseload midwife. The aim of this was to obtain a detailed description of the 36-week birth talk, and how it is delivered to, and perceived by, women and their birth partners. It would have been difficult to only ask midwives or women about this, as the answers would have missed a lot of the detail, so observations were made on five talks and then phenomenological interviews used to talk with the midwives, the women and their birth partners to answer the question on perceptions of the talk. This is also a good example of *triangulation*, that is, the use of more than one data collection tool to increase the validity of the results.

STRUCTURED OBSERVATION

The next two sections will look first at the use of structured observations, followed in the next section by the use of unstructured observation. In structured or systematic observation, data are often recorded on a checklist observation sheet that itemises the kinds of activities to be observed. The researcher will indicate, often with a tick, each time one of the items on the list occurs, for example, a checklist of the times in an antenatal group setting a midwife asks a direct question as a way of gaining involvement from those present. The results are usually presented numerically, in the form of the number of occasions (*frequency distribution*), a percentage, or displayed in a table or figure such as a bar chart. Polit and Beck (2008: 433) suggest:

> Structured observation involves the collection of observational data using formal instruments and protocols that dictate what to observe, how long to observe it, and how to record the intended information.

The items or variables to be recorded need clear and unambiguous *concept definitions*, that is, a precise description of its meaning or form to ensure accuracy of recording, especially where there are a number of observers involved. This helps to reduce the problem of the observer having to make a large number of inferences regarding an item such as 'gives emotional support'. What exactly does that mean in terms of what would be observed? The greater the degree of inference required, the less reliable the outcome. The ideal type of item for checklist observation includes those capable of being explicitly defined so that there is no question in the mind of the observer as to whether or not they have been identified.

As events and activities unfold so quickly, there is a limit to the number of different aspects the researcher can observe at once. Care has to be taken to avoid the checklist becoming too complex. For example, it may not be possible to accurately record the type, duration and form of touch between a midwife and woman in labour, as well as the duration of eye contact, and any additional non-verbal forms of interaction.

Not only should the optimum number of elements be considered in the checklist, but also the form of recording must be simplified to enable speed and accuracy. Simple ticks or crosses are the best form of recording items. Before using a checklist, the researcher should thoroughly practice with a pilot study. This may suggest ways of reducing the complexity of the list, as well as providing the researcher with an opportunity to develop the skill of observing and recording at the same time.

The limitation of an observational checklist is the depth of information that can be achieved, and the limited complexity of interactions that can be accurately observed. This type of approach is also restricted to predicted behaviour, and does not cope well with unexpected activities not included on the checklist. This means this form of observation is not appropriate where the researcher knows little about what will be observed (Polit and Beck 2008).

UNSTRUCTURED OBSERVATIONS

In contrast to the checklist approach of structured observation are the unstructured methods found in qualitative studies. This means that the researcher records in a more open and flowing way the events and behaviours they 'see'. Anthropologists and sociologists first developed this form of observation to examine the actions and interactions of people in their natural social world. One helpful description of researchers using this type of observation method is provided by Polit and Beck (2008: 402), who say:

> The aim of their research is to understand the behaviors and experiences of people as they actually occur in naturalistic settings. Qualitative researchers seek to observe people and their environments with a minimum of structure and interference.

One frequently used typology of observer roles when carrying out data collection was developed by Gold (1958) cited in Holloway and Wheeler (2010). This can be seen in Box 11.1. The different roles vary in the extent to which the researcher becomes directly involved with those observed, that is, whether the role is participant or non-participant. A further variation is the extent to which the observed are aware that they are being watched. The term 'overt' signifies that those in the setting are aware of the observer's role, and 'covert' to situations where they do not know that observation is taking place. Most health care research now takes the overt approach as there are considerable ethical issues raised by the concealment of data collection, as in covert

> **BOX 11.1 Gold's typology of observer role**
>
> Complete participant
> Participant as observer
> Observer as participant
> Complete observer
>
> Reproduced from Holloway and Wheeler, 2010:111.

research where the individual has not given their informed consent to take part. This is despite the possible advantage of reducing the 'observer effect', that is, people changing their behaviour because they know they are being observed (Holloway and Wheeler 2010).

A classic example of unstructured observation is the ethnographic study by Hunt (Hunt and Symonds 1995), where Hunt observed the culture of two maternity units over a 6-month period. The aim of the study was to understand the culture, work practices and strategies of midwives. As with most ethnographic studies, the interpretation of the role of observer was not static. Hunt appears at times to take on the role of 'participant as observer'. This can be seen in the following passage.

> *The maternity unit was frequently very busy and the staff seemed happy to cast me in the role of someone who was an additional pair of hands with some inquisitive and quirky habits (note-taking, etc.) ... I was on the outside and on the inside at the same time, and never really 'at home'. The role is somewhere between stranger and friend.* (p. 46)

This kind of study illustrates the richness of data developed through ethnographic work. It contrasts with checklist observational studies in that the researcher is interested in more in-depth information that does not necessarily follow a clearly anticipated path. There is also a great emphasis on discovering the form of behaviour found in natural settings, such as a labour ward.

Perhaps in no other form of data collection do researchers have to consider so carefully their role as researcher, as they play a very visible role within the setting. This is illustrated by Hunt (Hunt and Symonds 1995:51) who at one point has to consider the consequence of answering the ward phone when it rings. She initially decides not to, as this may involve changing what would have taken place if she had not been there. There is also the danger that performing one activity will adversely affect the role of observer, so for instance she comments:

> *I did not feel I was capable of being a full-time ethnographer and full-time telephonist.*

Hunt even carefully chooses the clothes she will wear as a researcher, deciding in the early stages to wear a white coat, and comments that:

> *For someone in a white coat it appeared that access was unrestricted.* (p. 45)

Later this is abandoned once people in the setting are used to her presence, as she felt there was an element of deception in being mistaken for someone 'medical'. The style of dress can have a profound effect on the way people may react in a situation to a researcher. These are not, therefore, trivial details, but are important elements the researcher has included in an attempt to demonstrate credibility, and to share with the reader the nature of the researcher's presence in the research environment.

RECORDING IN OBSERVATIONAL STUDIES

One issue for the observational researcher is how to record the observations. Checklist designs are easiest to imagine, as the observer uses pre-printed sheets consisting of columns or tables of items in which a tick is placed if an activity or event is observed. Where a study involves a number of observers, inter-observer reliability has to be demonstrated, that is, ensuring that the same event or item is recorded in the same way by each person carrying out the observations. This is where the training of observers plays a vital role in achieving consistency between observers (Watson et al. 2010).

Qualitative observational methods are more complex, and raise greater issues for the researcher. Field notes are the major form of recording observations in qualitative studies. These are narrative accounts of events and situations and can be made while activities are in progress, or they can be written up some time later. Each alternative has its advantages. The researcher may draw attention to themselves if they write their observations during events; however, there is a greater dependency on the accuracy of memory where notes are written up later. The method chosen will depend on the many factors that researchers find in a setting, although the tendency is to make at least some rough notes at the time and to develop these later.

Hunt (Hunt and Symonds 1995: 47) illustrates how she tackled this issue in her study. The aim in the following description is to allow the reader to feel as though they are in the setting and can follow the way in which the data are generated:

> My data collection took a variety of forms. The main activity was the production of field notes. During the visit I would use my notebook to record headings and key phrases that would help me in the recording. I also used the Dictaphone, usually in the toilet or store cupboard, to record key phrases and prompts. After each visit, when I returned home, I would write detailed field notes on the events of that visit. These were initially filed in date order. The field notes would include details of events and accounts of conversations. Much of the time was spent observing and informal interviewing those who had emerged as key informants. These interviews were unstructured and in the early days I recorded as much as possible of what was said, how it was said, to whom and on what occasions. The field notes also include lengthy descriptions of the labour ward, the office, the admission room, etc.

This description provides a comprehensive example of how recording is achieved in a qualitative observational study. Unfortunately, the more recently published studies using observation do not contain this wealth of detail.

ADVANTAGES OF OBSERVATION

Observation is the most appropriate way of collecting research data in many situations, as the researcher is able to see what actually happens, and does not depend on reports that may be distorted by memory or perception. In other words, they record what people actually do as opposed to what they say they do (Watson et al. 2010). In checklist studies, the frequency of events can be quantified, and relationships and correlation can be established.

It is in the area of qualitative research that observation can be particularly appropriate to midwifery research. Holloway and Wheeler (2010) point out that they are particularly useful in providing a holistic view of a setting and suggest that health professionals as observers have an advantage as insider as they can ask the kinds of questions that would not occur to an outsider. However, it is possible to argue the reverse of this, where an outsider may ask questions that the insider would not think to ask due to familiarity with the setting. The important point is that as observation takes place in a natural setting, it can provide an accurate picture of what actually happens. It can also take into account quite a large canvas of activity in the form of a description of, for example, a birth spread over a long time period. Qualitative observation also provides flexibility, in that the focus of attention can change as a result of early observations.

Observational studies are not frequently found in midwifery, although they clearly have much to offer in gaining answers to questions that are not amenable to other forms of data collection. As with interviews, they can be used in both a quantitative and qualitative approach, and appear to be extremely suitable for midwifery research either as a single method or in conjunction with other forms of data collection.

DISADVANTAGES OF OBSERVATION

Despite the positive aspects of this method, there are a number of pitfalls. Ethical problems are a major concern for the qualitative researcher, especially where covert observation is being used. The issue is one of observing individuals who have not given their permission to be included in a study. This goes against the basic principles of informed consent discussed in Chapter 8.

However, one of the difficulties in observation is the problem of *reactivity*, when people who are told what is being observed may change their normal behaviour and so distort the accuracy of the results. Take, for instance, the example given in Chapter 8 of observing student midwives' hand-washing techniques and imagine indicating to a student that their technique is about to be observed. The result may be that their technique is surprisingly good but may be far from an accurate picture of normal activity!

The question of ethics is also raised in situations where the observer sees an activity that may put individuals at risk, or is an unprofessional act carried out by a member of staff. Although the researcher tries to maintain a confidential relationship with subjects, in certain circumstances it is not possible to honour this. One example would be where the observer has a public duty to disclose information, as in the case of observing unlawful or unprofessional activity or something that may potentially put a child at risk. In such situations the researcher is obliged to report these observations, and must abandon the researcher role for that of the midwife (see Chapter 8 for a discussion of these issues).

From a practical point of view, observation is a very time consuming and therefore an expensive method. It also requires a great deal of interpersonal skills on the part of the observer, who should have training and experience with this method. Where more than one person is involved with the data gathering, there is also the problem of inter-observer reliability. This concerns the extent to which different observers select, interpret and record events in different ways.

One of the most obvious problems already referred to is that of *reactivity*, where people act differently because they know they are part of a research study. This seems an inevitable feature of observations made in the early stages of a study, or in early interactions with individuals. A similar situation is recorded by Hunt (Hunt and Symonds 1995: 46):

> *During the early fieldwork stages (the first two or three weeks) it was clear that the staff were making a very special effort to be good communicators. One midwife asked if I would tape her as she encouraged or coached a woman in the second stage of labour. It was an outstanding, energetic performance, worthy of its tape-recording and the language will be familiar to many midwives ... The performance seemed to call for an applause, and the midwife smiled and seemed almost to bow at the end. She asked if that was what my research was all about. She explained she thought she was a good communicator and I should put this in my research. I promised I would.*

This extract raises the issue of validity. The observer has to consider the extent to which the observations are a true picture of what is going on. The 'ironic' tone of the authors' description indicates that it is usually clear to the researcher when observations are not a true reflection of activities. This challenge to both the reliability of the method and validity of the results is reduced where the observation extends over a longer time period, where people relax more into their usual way of behaving.

A further problem for the midwife researcher is the difficulty of being able to stand back from the familiar taken-for-granted routine of the maternity setting, and ask, 'why do things happen like this?' In anthropological terms, this is called establishing *'cultural strangeness'*, where the aim is to see things from an outsider's point of view. The longer the researcher is in the field setting, however, the greater the danger of what is referred to as *'going native'*. This term also comes from anthropological studies where, over an extended period of observing tribes, researchers would become so at home with the new culture that they would stop seeing activities and customs as 'strange' or noteworthy. In qualitative research, it refers to the researcher becoming over-familiar with the research setting and no longer noticing the kind of elements that need to be included in the observations. This results in a loss of objectivity and observations become subject to researcher bias (Polit and Beck 2008).

A major problem for researchers is one of selectivity. As it is not possible to observe everything that is going on, or see things from every angle, decisions have to be made on where observers will place themselves, and what they will attempt to observe. This will inevitably lead to some things being observed and others left out. In the same way, it is not possible to record everything, and some details will be omitted. Wood and Ross-Kerr (2006: 172) warn that no two observers will observe the same things or observe in the same way, which illustrates that observation is open to some variation and in its 'open' form will, at least to some extent, by influenced by the observer. In some situations there is also the possibility of misinterpreting what is going on. This is particularly true when observing a long-established relationship where subtle patterns of communication styles have been developed and understood between people. These can appear strange or alien to the observer. The difference between cajoling someone to do something and apparently being hostile or unsympathetic can easily be misinterpreted by the researcher unaware of the usual pattern of conversation between people.

Observer bias is a further concern, where researchers may be inclined to look out for certain activities and ignore others that do not fit in with their views or expectations. Where each period of observation is lengthy, *observer drift* or what Mcilfatrick (2008: 315) refers to as *'observer fatigue'* can also be a problem, where observers lose concentration after a time, and finds themselves thinking of other things, and lose awareness of what is happening. This will clearly affect the quality and accuracy of the data (Griffiths and Rafferty 2010). In some situations, time sampling is carried out so that the observation period is broken down into shorter segments and the researcher attempts to sample across all the time periods. This allows the researcher to remain relatively fresh throughout the period of observation. Where the researcher is concentrating on events, such as a birth, this is not always a viable alternative, and an awareness of the danger of observer drift is the only precaution possible.

This range of possible pitfalls illustrates the complexity of this method. A number of excellent examples of qualitative research using observation exist in midwifery (e.g. Hunt and Symonds 1995, Davies 1996), which help the novice researcher to be aware of the problems.

CONDUCTING RESEARCH

As with each of the methods of research covered so far, the researcher must ensure that observation is the appropriate choice for the study aim. In situations where self-reports may be inaccurate, or where there is a need to consider a holistic view, then observation may be the best method.

The decision on which type of observation should be used is based on the requirements of the research question. Where the question relates to a quantification of results, such as 'how often' or 'how much', or where the question is related to establishing whether something happens or not and with what frequency, a checklist design will be appropriate. This will take the form of a structured sheet that looks like a spreadsheet or grid, to allow ease of completion in the form of ticks, code numbers, or letters.

Where the research question does not imply a quantitative approach, but is more concerned with developing a broad understanding of how people act in a natural setting, as in an ethnographic study, then a participant or non-participant observation study should be designed.

The exact role the researcher will play in this kind of research will require thought. The variation in role from participant to non-participant observer should be considered (see Box 11.1). This does not necessarily mean that the researcher will stay within one role. The consequences of the different types of researcher role, however, must be considered in relation to their influence on those observed and the consequence for the data gathered.

At an early point, the ethical implications of the study need to be considered. Where an ethics committee (LREC) is involved, informed consent and the issue of possible deception should be addressed in a way that will satisfy the committee that consent has been considered, and harm will be avoided.

There are a large number of skills required of the observer. Hunt (Hunt and Symonds 1995: 40) elaborates on the skills required in an ethnographic study by saying:

> *Ethnography makes use of basic skills such as listening, watching, asking questions and the skills of 'sussing out'.*

By this she means that researchers have to work out what is going on in a situation without using their own stereotypes and preconceptions. Rather, they should try and see things through the eyes of those observed. In terms of the practical activities concerned, researchers must decide on the issues of what to record, and how. It is important in observation to have clear concept definitions for the items that will be recorded. This is true of checklist observation, as well as qualitative observational approaches.

The how of recording will depend on the extent to which contemporary recording may disrupt the flow of activities being observed. The main alternatives will be note taking at the time or some time later, or the use of an audio recorder. The exact details of what is recorded will change during the course of observation. Early notes may be very broad, and will try to establish some ideas of the kind of pattern of activity taking place. They will then become more focused, depending on earlier observations and the questions arising from the field notes. Hunt (Hunt and Symonds 1995: 48) provides an insight into the content of early field notes as follows:

> *The field notes were generally descriptive accounts of events observed in the field. Direct quotations were included whenever possible as were descriptions of such aspects as the tone of voice and the body language of the contributor. The field notes also included sketches of some aspects of the environment and maps to remind me of the layout of the unit.*

The analysis stage of this kind of data is a very sophisticated activity. As with the analysis of quantitative data, advice and help should be sought from those with previous experience. In presenting the qualitative report or article, the structure is very different from that of a quantitative report or article. Some of the sources of work referred to in this chapter should be considered as a guide for writing the report in order to do full justice to the information collected.

CRITIQUING RESEARCH

In critiquing observational research articles, we have to decide whether this was a suitable method to answer the research question. It is important to determine what the researcher was observing and how. In both checklist and qualitative approaches, does the researcher give a clear concept definition for the items being observed?

Perhaps only second to experimental design, observation raises a number of ethical issues, so an important element it to ensure that an ethics committee approves the study. Was the research overt or covert, that is, were people aware that they were being observed or not? Was permission sought from subjects where it was overt? Where permission was not sought, does the researcher provide a convincing justification for not securing this?

Where the researcher is present in the research setting, as opposed to the use of cameras, we must consider the extent to which the researcher may have had an influence on the people and events observed. What did the researcher do to try to minimise the reactive effect on subjects? In good qualitative studies, we should expect researchers to provide a clear description of how they presented themselves in the setting in terms of dress and behaviour. Do the researchers appear to display any bias, emotions, and prejudices in their dealings with those observed which may have influenced the quality of the data collected? Do the researchers appear to gravitate towards certain people in the study, and avoid others? In other words, has there been a bias in who was observed that might have produced untypical results?

Where more than one observer was responsible for the data collection, how was inter-observer reliability achieved? Even where there is only one observer, it is important to establish if any training was received or a pilot study undertaken.

Has the researcher included other methods of data collections such as structured or unstructured interviews, or the use of diaries, or other form of documentary methods? Is the interplay between the different methods explained? In unstructured observation, the researcher using a qualitative approach should have produced, 'thick' or 'rich' data. Does this enhance credibility so it almost feels as if you are there?

When it comes to analysis, do the researchers leave a decision trail so that you can audit the way they have moved through the data collection to the establishment of the categories used to present the findings? Overall, do the researchers convince you that they have tried to be as rigorous as possible throughout the study?

KEY POINTS

- Observation can be used to produce quantitative or qualitative data.
- Although it is not used as often as some of the other methods, it can play an important part in answering important questions in a holistic and woman-centred way.
- In observation, the main issues concern the degree of structure in the data collection and the influence of the observer's presence on what is observed.
- There are a large number of decisions to make prior to the study by researchers. These include the nature of the role they will play, the amount of interaction they will have with those observed, the method of recording, the extent of recording, and the method of analysis.
- The time period needed for some studies makes this a costly method of collecting data, and one that requires a large amount of personal skills, as well as research expertise. The benefits of such an approach, however, are considerable.

REFERENCES

Davies, R., 1996. 'Practitioners in their own right': an ethnographic study of the perceptions of student midwives'. In: Robinson, S., Thomson, A. (Eds.), Midwives, Research and Childbirth, vol. 4. Chapman and Hall, London.

Griffiths, P., Rafferty, A.M., 2010. Outcome measures. In: Gerrish, K., Lacey, A. (Eds.), The Research Process in Nursing, sixth ed. Wiley-Blackwell, Chichester.

Holloway, I., Wheeler, S., 2010. Qualitative Research for Nurses, third ed. Wiley-Blackwell, Chichester.

Hunt, S., Symonds, A., 1995. The Social Meaning of Midwifery. Macmillan, Houndmills.

Kemp, J., Sandall, J., 2010. Normal birth, magical birth: the role of the 36-week birth talk in caseload midwifery practice. Midwifery 26 (2), 211–221.

Mcilfatrick, S., 2008. Observation. In: Watson, R., McKenna, H., Cowman, S., Keady, J. (Eds.), Nursing Research: Designs and Methods. Churchill Livingstone, Edinburgh.

Polit, D., Beck, C., 2008. Nursing Research: Generating and Assessing Evidence for Nursing Practice, eighth ed. Lippincott Williams and Wilkins, Philadelphia.

Watson, H., Booth, J., Whyte, R., 2010. Observation. In: Gerrish, K., Lacey, A. (eds.), The Research Process in Nursing, sixth ed. Wiley-Blackwell, Chichester.

Wood, M., Ross-Kerr, J., 2006. Basic Steps in Planning Nursing Research: From Question to Proposal, sixth ed. Jones and Bartlett, Sudbury.

Experiments

12

Evidence-based practice has increased the demand for research that can unambiguously demonstrate the best options for clinical care. Experimental design has established itself as the most widely recognised and respected source of such evidence. In medicine, the experiment frequently takes the form of the randomised control trial (**RCT**). This method of collecting research data has become so powerful in determining the effectiveness of treatments that it is used by some as a measure against which all other methods are compared. As many clinical procedures in maternity care are influenced by experimental research, it is crucial that midwives can evaluate such studies and not accept them without question.

The purpose of this chapter is to consider the basic principles of experimental design, and to recognise the strengths, as well as the limitations, of this approach. As experiments can be designed in a number of ways, the chapter will also outline some of these various forms.

WHY ARE EXPERIMENTS SPECIAL?

Experiments are highly regarded in health care and have been traditionally associated with the idea of 'scientific method'. This may be due to the belief that they are more accurate or 'objective' than other forms of data collection. This has led to their prominent position in 'hierarchies of evidence' that attempt to indicate the most reliable sources of information. The result is that hierarchies 'privilege' the RCT in a way that makes them the main source of knowledge within medicine (Spiby and Munro 2010).

Why do experimental designs have such a high status in health care, particularly in regard to evidence-based practice? The answer lies in what they can achieve and the characteristics they possess. Firstly, they have provided the basis on which a great deal of our current health care knowledge and theory has been based, especially in the form of the randomised control trial. RCTs, according to Burns and Grove (2009), provide the strongest research evidence for practice. This is because they examine the likelihood of a cause-and-effect relationship between variables through the use of statistical calculations. Such calculations determine the extent to which the results of an experiment could have happened by chance and is indicated by the 'p' value. This takes the form

© 2011 Elsevier Ltd. All rights reserved.

BOX 12.1 Probability values

Probability values indicate the extent to which the difference in the results between two groups could have happened by chance. The 'p' stands for 'probability'. This translates into how many times out of a hundred, or even a thousand, the difference between two groups of data could happen purely by chance. The smaller the likelihood that a difference could have happened by chance, the more certain we can be that the experiment has demonstrated a cause-and-effect relationship. In other words, the intervention does produce the desired effect.

The value of 'p' is expressed as a decimal, and has to be converted to a fraction to work out the element of chance. Take the example of '$p < 0.05$'. We first convert 0.05 to a fraction by drawing a line underneath the numbers so that they become the top line of the fraction; then put a '1' underneath the decimal point, and a '0' underneath every figure after the point. This may sound complicated, but if you write it out for yourself, 0.05 becomes 05/100. In other words, the likelihood of the difference between the results of two groups in the study happening purely by chance is less than 5 in 100 times. Or, put another way, 95 times out of 100 the effect you wanted will be produced by the intervention used in the study.

This figure of $p < 0.05$ is regarded as the minimum value that may suggest a relationship between the dependent and independent variable. Notice that there is still a margin of error. It does not mean that one thing definitely causes the other; the results would have happened purely by chance 5 in 100 times. This means that for 95% of the time you can be satisfied that a cause-and-effect relationship does exist.

The most frequently used values to indicate probability are as follows:

P value	Probability of difference happening by chance
< 0.05	less than 5 in 100
< 0.01	less than 1 in 100
< 0.001	less than 1 in 1000
NS	non-significant (i.e. the probability that chance is responsible for the result is so large that a 'p' value is not used).

It is recommended that you consult a statistics book for more information.

of decimal number often found in or under a table of results or in the text of a research article. It is reasonably easy to interpret this once you are familiar with the basic idea underpinning probability (see Box 12.1).

CHARACTERISTICS OF EXPERIMENTAL DESIGN

What are the essential features of an experiment? Unlike other methods (apart from action research), the experiment is a form of research where the researcher is active in the situation and not just a gatherer of information. The researcher makes something happen and is responsible for controlling the way that something is introduced into the situation. So a common form of the experiment is where there are two groups of participants and the researcher will introduce an intervention to one group but not the other and then see if

> **BOX 12.2 Example of a randomised control trial of extended midwifery support (EMS) on the duration of breastfeeding (McDonald et al. 2010)**
>
> The aim of this Australian RCT set in a large public teaching hospital was to evaluate the effects of an extended midwifery support (EMS) programme on the proportion of women who breastfeed fully to 6 months. The sample consisted of 849 women who consented to take part in the study. Participants must have given birth to a healthy, term, singleton baby and wished to breastfeed. The women were allocated at random to either the extended support group (independent variable), where they were offered a one-to-one postnatal educational session and weekly home visits with additional telephone contact by a midwife until their baby was 6 weeks old, or to the standard postnatal midwifery support group (control). The women were first stratified for parity and education level. The main outcome measures (dependent variables) were the prevalence of full and any breastfeeding at 6 months postpartum. The results showed that there was no difference between the groups at 6 months postpartum for either full breastfeeding or any breastfeeding. The researchers concluded that the EMS programme did not succeed in improving breastfeeding rates in a setting where there was already a high initiation of breastfeeding.

those in the experimental group have a different outcome to those in the control group. See Box 12.2 for an example.

According to Burns and Grove (2009: 262), the three elements that confirm a study as a true experiment are:

- randomisation,
- researcher-controlled manipulation of the independent variable (the experimental variable),
- researcher control of the experimental situation, including a control or comparison group.

Together, these three elements help to rule out alternative ways of explaining a particular outcome to a study other than the variable introduced by the researcher. Each of these elements will now be examined.

RANDOMISATION

Randomisation is a term that may apply to both the sampling procedure used in a study (see Chapter 14), and the allocation of individuals to an experimental (sometimes called intervention) or control group. Random sampling occurs when every member of a study population (all those with the relevant characteristics, such as those going home from a midwifery-led unit over a 3-month period) has an equal chance of being included in the study. This is not easy to achieve in a total group, as individuals must first agree to take part in a clinical study; it is not simply a case of picking them out of a population and expecting them to accept a form of intervention allocated to them. In most cases, randomisation refers to *random assignment* or *random allocation*. This is the process of allocating participants to either the experimental or control group in a random manner *once they have agreed to take part in the study*. In other words, an individual entering the study should be allocated to a treatment or intervention group in a way that ensures they have an equal chance of being in either group. The exact method used to randomise those in a study will be explained in Chapter 14. It is a very precise and methodical system and it not 'haphazard', which is a misunderstanding of the term.

The purpose of randomisation is to reduce the possibility of bias where people with certain characteristics that might affect the outcome are unevenly distributed between the two groups in a study. The implication of this is that the groups would initially differ from each other, which would make it impossible to rule out the influence of factors built in to the characteristics of those in the two groups. Nelson et al. (2010) support this by stating that experiments are based on the assumption that the groups were similar at the start of the experiment before anything is introduced. If they differ at the end, then it is easier to argue that the difference is due to the experimental variable. Randomisation also ensures that additional factor, called *'confounding variables'*, that may also influence the results are evenly distributed between the two groups. In other words, randomisation should allow the researcher to compare like with like.

In experimental design, the existence of a comparison group that does not receive the independent variable is crucial. The role of the control group is to act as a comparison by establishing what the typical outcome would be if the experimental variable had not been introduced. In evidence-based practice, this is important in deciding whether an intervention would make any difference to the outcome? The control group theoretically remains the same over the experimental period, as they do not receive the treatment or intervention that forms the independent variable. This allows the investigator to reduce the effect of what has variously been called the *'attention factor'*, or the *'Hawthorne effect'* (this will be explained in more detail later in this chapter). These terms relate to a phenomenon where individuals report a change influenced by their participation in a study. In other words, a change in the dependent variable may be due to a feeling of being 'special' and which produces a reaction that 'mimics' a real change.

Not all studies have a separate control group. One group can receive two interventions in turn, for example, a conventional approach followed by an experimental approach. In this way, individuals act as their own control (Nelson et al. 2010). It is also possible for two separate groups to receive the same two interventions, but in a different order. Here again, they are acting as their own controls in that they receive both interventions and rule out the possibility that any differences are the result of varying characteristics of those in the two groups. This kind of approach is referred to as a *cross-over design study*.

MANIPULATION

The second feature of experimental design is manipulation, which means the experimenter manipulates or introduces the independent variable, usually an intervention or treatment to the experimental group, but withholds it from the control group who receive either an alternative, or nothing (Polit and Beck 2008). In the words of Smith (2008), if there is no intervention introduced by the researcher then there is no experiment! In the example in Box 12.2, the researchers made available to one group extended midwifery support in the form of a one-to-one postnatal educational session, weekly home visits and additional telephone contact by a midwife until their baby was 6 weeks old, while the control group had routine care.

CONTROL

Control is the final feature of experimental design, where the researcher reduces the possible effect of other independent variables on the outcome measure of the study. This means that the experimenter must have the ability to control not only the independent variable but also other elements within the experimental setting that might make a difference to the dependent variable (outcome measure). For example, they must ensure that everyone in the study has an equal chance of being in the experimental group (random allocation). If this is achieved, then the researcher can say that they have controlled for extraneous factors that may influence the dependent variable. In the study in Box 12.2., the researchers controlled for parity and educational level, which might have had an impact on the outcome by first putting the group into parity and education subgroups and randomly choosing from each group so that these factors were equalised through the design of the study

It is the researcher's ability to achieve maximum control that illustrates the degree of rigour in the study. This includes control over the way any interventions are provided. All procedures must be applied in exactly the same way to each individual so that consistency is achieved and other possible explanations for differences in outcomes eliminated. Measurements of the dependent variable should also be under the control of the researcher. The measuring instrument should be accurate and consistent, and where more than one person is involved in the measurement, the researcher should ensure that everyone is measuring in the same way. This is called *inter-rater reliability*.

Taken together, we can see all three features of an experiment make extraordinary demands on the skills and power of the researcher and make experiments a very complex form of research.

Blinding

Before moving on, there are two important aspects of control in medical or obstetric research that need to be highlighted, as they are becoming more important in assessing the rigour of those experimental designs with clinical interventions and objectively measured outcomes. These are *allocation concealment* and *blinding*. At the start of a study, as individuals are being allocated to the experimental or control group, it is essential that those carrying out the allocation cannot anticipate the group to which the next person will be allocated. This is so they do not tamper with who goes where, on the basis of their knowledge of what the person might receive. *Blinding* or *masking* means that those in the study do not know the intervention or treatment an individual has received. This is an attempt to maintain the objectivity of the method by protecting the results from the accusation that they are inaccurate as they have been spoilt or compromised by poor design. Using sealed envelopes so that it is not possible to anticipate the allocation until the envelope has been opened is frequently used in clinical trials to avoid the problem of allocation concealment. Blinding is more complicated and involves more people, as the risk of bias can come from several sources. It involves the risk of people acting differently if they know to which group the individual has been allocated during the course of a clinical trial. Smith (2008) suggests that if masking is not carried out adequately there is an increased chance that measurement estimates can be subconsciously raised in favour of the experimental intervention. Single blinding is where either the person receiving an intervention or the person measuring the outcome is shielded from knowing whether the individual was in the experimental or control group. Double blinding is where both the study individual and those providing care or measuring the outcome are unaware to which group the individual was allocated.

Taken together, the two aspects of allocation concealment and blinding are amongst the most important aspects of clinical RCTs, as they can have a drastic effect on the accuracy of the outcome in trials. In relation to nursing and midwifery research, although control is an important aspect, concealment and blinding is not always sensible or possible, as the intervention may be difficult to hide from those receiving it and those involved in the care, for example spending time in water in labour, or receiving food in labour. This difficulty in blinding is a consequence of variations in the way research is conducted in different health care areas where constraints on the levels of control are inevitable and not necessarily a weakness in design.

This is clear in the example in Box 12.2. The outcome measurements are collected through a self-report questionnaire and diary kept by participants in the study. There were no objective measures or assessments by a member of the research team. Women clearly were aware of whether they received additional support in the form of visits and phone calls or not. In this way, the study is a demonstration of the variations in the way RCTs are conducted and how interventions and measurements in midwifery research can vary from those in medical or obstetric research.

THE HYPOTHESIS

Wood and Ross-Kerr (2006) categorise the experiment as a level-three research question (see Chapter 2). To achieve this level, they suggest that the researcher should be able to predict what will happen (have a hypothesis), and provide a theory based on previous research findings to explain it. One of the chief purposes of the experiment, then, is to test a hypothesis and so establish causality, that is, one variable is capable of causing or bringing about a direct effect on another variable. The researcher should state the hypothesis at the start of the study. This statement can take two forms: *the research or scientific hypothesis* and the *null-hypothesis* (also called a *statistical hypothesis*). The research hypothesis states the predicted difference in outcomes between the two groups. It usually contains words such as *'more than', 'higher'* or *'less than' or 'lower'*, whichever indicates a better outcome. The null-hypothesis predicts that there will be no difference between the two groups (see Chapter 7); in other words, the intervention will not affect the outcome. This is the situation in the study by

O'sullivan et al. (2009), who believed that allowing women to have something light to eat during labour would not affect major clinical outcomes, which the data supported. In this case, the most favourable result would be no difference in outcome between the group who received only water and the group allowed light food.

For those unfamiliar with hypotheses, it is not always easy to work out which is the dependent and which is the independent variable in the statement of the hypothesis. One helpful method of distinguishing between the two is to identify which comes first chronologically and which comes or is measured last. The item that comes last is the dependent variable (the effect), and the item that comes first is the independent variable (the cause). So, in the case of O'sullivan et al. (2009) just mentioned on eating in labour, the items measured last would be the clinical outcomes of the birth, these included spontaneous vaginal birth rate, duration of labour, need for augmentation of labour, instrumental and Caesarean birth rates, incidence of vomiting, and neonatal outcome. Each of those would be a dependent variable (as an RCT can have more than one dependent variable). What came before them in time was eating the food, so that is the independent variable. Box 12.3 provides some examples of hypotheses and illustrates the dependent and independent variables in each case. In each of the examples in the box, identify what chronologically would have to be measured first. This will be the independent variable; the last item to be measured will be the dependent variable. Look what happens in the null-hypothesis example.

TYPES OF EXPERIMENTS

Experimental design can take a number of alternative forms. Often these variations relate to a second 'control' group and how people are allocated to them, and also variations in the point at which measurements take place. The classic

---

BOX 12.3 Examples of research hypotheses and a null-hypothesis

- The assumption (*hypothesis*) that additional postnatal support, in the form of telephone calls and home visits by a midwife (*independent variable*), would be beneficial for the duration of breastfeeding (*dependent variable*) was tested (McDonald et al. 2010). *Research hypothesis*
- Women who attended the 'Having a Baby' programme (*independent variable*) would have higher perceived parenting self-efficacy and knowledge scores(*dependent variable*), and lower baby worry scores 8 weeks after the birth(*dependent variable*), compared with those who attended the regular programme (*control*). It was also hypothesised that there would be no difference in labour (*dependent variable*) and birth outcomes (*dependent variable*) (Svensson et al. 2009). *Research hypothesis*
- The null-hypothesis was that there would be no difference in breastfeeding duration at 6 and 17 weeks (*dependent variable*), between 'a hands off' positioning and attachment intervention at first postnatal ward feed by midwives (*independent variable*) and routine care (*control*) (Wallace et al. 2006). *Null-hypothesis.*

writers on the subject, Campbell and Stanley (1963), suggested that there were three main variations:

- the pre-test post-test control group,
- the post-test only design,
- the Solomon four-group design.

THE PRE-TEST POST-TEST CONTROL GROUP

This is the most commonly used and perhaps the best known design, where subjects are randomly allocated to the experimental or control group (Polit and Beck 2008). The idea is to have two balanced groups in terms of the personal attributes that might make a difference to the outcome. Both groups are measured in relation to an outcome measure (dependent variable) prior to any intervention, and this acts as a base-line measurement. At this point these measurements should confirm that the two groups are comparable. In the intervention phase, the experimental group receives the new intervention, whilst the control group receives either the current or no intervention/treatment (although they may receive a placebo). Following this phase, both groups are retested or measured again, and any differences subjected to statistical analysis. This calculates the extent to which any differences between the two groups at the end could be due to chance, and not the result of the experimental intervention (Figure 12.1).

This method can be carried out using two different groups measured over the same time period, or a single group using a cross-over design (see above). This allows those in the study to act as their own controls. The first approach using two different groups is known as an *unrelated, between,* or *different subject* design, and the second a *related, within* or *same subject* design. It is worth considering that where one group receives both interventions, there can be a *'carry-over'* effect, where benefits from the first treatment may still influence the individual once exposed to the second intervention. To reduce this possibility, the order of the interventions is frequently randomised for those in the group.

POST-TEST ONLY DESIGN

A problem with the pre-test post-test design is that measuring the groups before an intervention is not always possible. There is also the problem that the first measurement may sensitise the subjects in such a way that they perform better on the second occasion because of the experience gained as a result of the first measurement. The post-test only design (Figure 12.2) is an

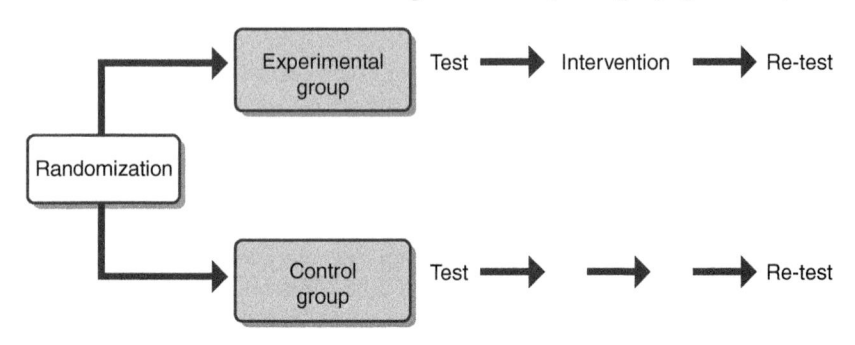

FIG 12.1 The pre-test, post-test design.

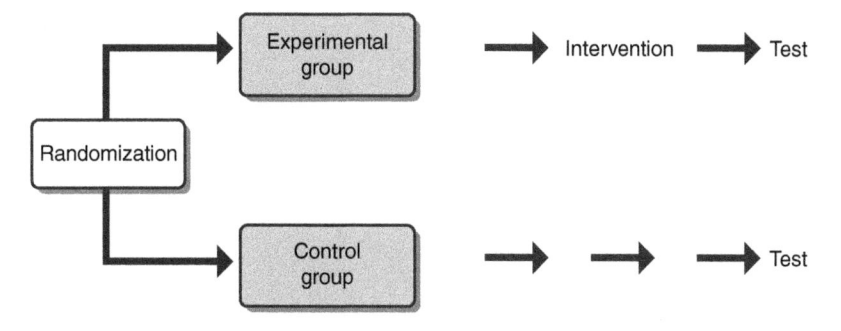

FIG 12.2 The post-test only design test.

attempt to reduce this familiarity effect by only measuring the variables at the end of the experiment. The limitation of this design is that it is not possible to say whether the two groups were similar at the start of the study. The difference in measurement could have been due to characteristics existing within the groups before the intervention.

SOLOMON FOUR-GROUP DESIGN

In order to overcome the disadvantages of both the previous examples, the Solomon four-group design has been developed. As can be seen from Figure 12.3, this is really a combination of both the previous designs. This means that as well as being able to eliminate the disadvantage of an after-only design, the effect of pre-testing can be assessed.

The immediate problem is one of gaining a sufficient number of people for all four groups. In addition, the possibility of some people dropping out (*subject mortality* or *subject attrition*) is even greater with this number of participants. The researcher may no longer be comparing like with like if the numbers in some of the groups have changed during the study period. This kind of design is very complex to organise and, naturally, very costly. Overall, we can see that this is a large-scale design that requires a great deal of time, resources and expertise.

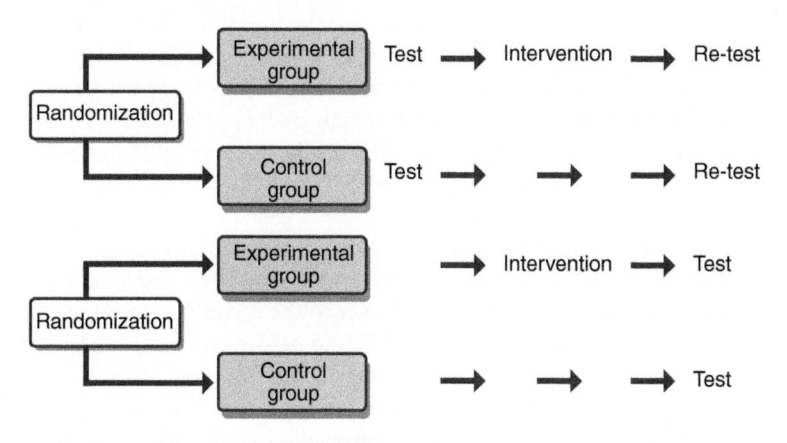

FIG 12.3 The Solomon four-group design.

12 THREATS TO VALIDITY

Although experimental designs are held in high regard, their use does not guarantee accuracy as there are a number of reasons why the results of an experiment may be inaccurate. The classic work of Campbell and Stanley (1963) still provides the best summary of these problems, usually referred to as 'threats to validity'. These come in two types; those that relate to the experiment itself (*internal threats to validity*) and those that relate to generalising the results to other situations (*external threats to validity*).

According to Campbell and Stanley (1963), any of the following may result in a threat to internal validity; these are factors within a study that may lead to the researcher mistakenly concluding they have found a causal relationship between the dependent and independent variable:

- *History* (the effect of external events on study outcomes): In this situation it is not the study's independent variable that has influenced the outcome, but something outside the study, sometimes referred to as a *confounding variable*. For example, a health scare about artificial feeds, or publicity where a celebrity chooses an elective Caesarean section, may influence the behaviour, attitude or knowledge of those in a study. The impact of history may be mistaken for the influence of a study intervention.
- *Testing* (the effect that being observed or tested has on the study outcomes): This refers to the consequence of pre-testing on the results of a later retest. The first test may encourage an individual to think about issues that influence how they answer later in the post-test, e.g. accepting screening tests. Here, it is the influence of the first test and not the intervention that has made a difference to the results.
- *Instrumentation* (the extent to which the instrument used to gather information in the study is accurate): Instrumentation is where pre- and post-differences are due to the data collection instrument changing over time, or the skills or accuracy of the data gatherers changing over time. This may produce different results that are mistakenly interpreted as due to the independent variable, e.g. variations in weighing scale accuracy.
- *Maturation* (the effect of the passage of time on individuals in the sample): This relates to normal physical, psychological, and social changes that occur to individuals that are unrelated to the variables in the study. Over time, people physically change, adapt, develop new skills, change attitude and so on. This may result in a change between pre- and post-testing results. Maturation changes can also occur over shorter periods. Even in the course of a day, we can change physically, or develop insights that, if subjected to retesting, may suggest a change due to an intervention rather than a normally occurring event.
- *Regression* (a statistical phenomenon): This is a frequently observed situation in statistics where there is a tendency for extreme scores or measurements in a study to move closer to the mean (average) when repeated testing takes place. This relates to before and after measurements (pre-test/post-test).
- *Mortality* (the effect caused by people dropping out of a study before all the measurements have been made, also called *sample attrition*): Although

an experimental and control group may have been similar at the start of a study, those who decided to drop out of a study may share common characteristic such as age, parity, or being smokers. Those remaining are no longer quite as similar as those in the other group, so the researcher is no longer comparing like with like.
- *Interactive effects* (the extent to which each of these threats interacts to influence the outcome of a study): In the same way that the individual threats may influence those in one group rather than another, so the range of influences may be acting on all those selected and so influence the results.

The second area of threat is that of *external validity* and considers those factors that limit the extent to which findings can apply to other settings. There are three main threats that need to be considered, and these relate to:

- *Selection effects*: This relates to the people selected for inclusion in the study.
- *Reactive effects*: The factors relating to how people respond within the experiment.
- *Measurement effects*: The effect of measurement techniques on the results.

Selection effects refer to the extent to which the characteristics of the sample may not have been truly representative of the population, and so it is unwise to generalise from the results of this particular sample. For instance, in some experiments poor sampling methods may have resulted in women from a particular social class, age group, or parity being over-represented in the sample. This may have produced results that cannot be applied to all women.

The *reactive effect* is the way in which some people respond to being in an experimental situation. They may behave in ways that are influenced by feeling special, or by a desire to help the experimenter succeed or have positive results. In this situation the results are not really due to the independent variable.

This was found in a classic American study on motivation that looked at people working in the Hawthorne plant of an electricity company in Chicago. Although the study set out to examine the effect of heating and lighting and other environmental factors on output, it was found that whether these factors were raised or lowered, productivity increased. It was realised that it was not the heating or lighting affecting the output; it was the result of feeling special because they were receiving attention from the researchers that influenced their work level. This gave rise to the term '*Hawthorne effect*', mentioned earlier in this chapter, which relates to the reactive effect of being part of a study.

Finally, the *measurement effect* considers the effect of testing on those in a study. If we accept that pre-testing knowledge or attitude may influence retesting (due to people having an opportunity to reflect on how they feel about the subject of the test), then we have to acknowledge that testing may reduce the extent to which the results of the study can be applied to others. This is because following testing, those in the sample are no longer typical of other people, as they have experienced something, or reflected on topics or values, that now make them different from others who have not been exposed in the same way.

One further problem area relates to the experimenter. Bias may emerge where researchers, in their enthusiasm for the study, may subconsciously influence people in non-verbal ways, such as positive nods of the head, or smiling when certain answers are given. Similarly, those in the study may provide answers or try hard to carry out the wishes of the experimenter because they like the individual and want the study to be successful. Their reactions to the procedures may also be affected by their knowledge of whether they are in the experimental or control group. These problems can be reduced by means of blind and double-blind studies, discussed above.

QUASI-EXPERIMENTAL DESIGNS

Although experimental design is regarded as one of the strongest methods of establishing cause-and-effect relationships, it is not always possible to apply this approach in every situation. The reasons for this can be practical, such as difficulties in controlling the effect of other independent variables, or ethical, where it would not be acceptable to allocate people to an experimental and control group. For example, it would not be ethical to allocate some women to a Caesarean section group or a normal birth group, as this would take away choice and could disadvantage them. Similarly, it would not be possible to randomly allocate women to a smoking or non-smoking group to examine the consequence of smoking on the fetus.

Where it is not possible to meet the strict conditions of experiments, there are a number of near alternatives that can be used. The *quasi-experiment* is one such option. This looks very much like an experiment, often with an experimental and control group, and with the researcher introducing an intervention. In this kind of study those in each group are chosen to be as similar as possible (Norman and Humphrey 2008). It differs from a true experiment because it lacks either control, or randomisation. In most cases it is the lack of random allocation to the two groups that is missing. An example would be women on one maternity ward having sessions on relaxation to measure its effect on stress or anxiety, and those on a second ward being used as a control and not receiving the relaxation. This makes management of the research easier, as all those in one setting will receive the same approach. It also reduces the risk of 'contamination' where individuals may be influenced by what they see happening to those alongside them.

Unfortunately, having all those in one setting receiving the intervention, rather than random allocation, will weaken the extent to which we have compared like with like. Differences between those in the two groups could make a difference to the outcome. In the relaxation example, it could be that some women already practice yoga or meditation, or there could be differences in personality between women on the two wards.

For this reason, quasi-experimental studies are not as persuasive as a true experimental design as they contain many threats to internal validity (Schmidt and Brown 2009). It is possible to strengthen them by taking measurements of both groups prior to the intervention so that we can see the extent to which they are similar and so accept them as reasonably comparable. In research terms, this approach of two non-randomised groups is referred to as *non-equivalent control group design*. The result is that the studies can best be described as level-two studies (Wood and Ross-Kerr 2006) as they indicate correlation rather than cause and effect.

EX POST FACTO STUDIES

In quasi-experimental design, although randomisation was not achieved, the researcher still introduced an independent variable into the situation, exposing the experimental group to the intervention but not the control group. In some situations, not only is it difficult to carry out randomisation, but it can also be difficult to introduce the independent variable. In this situation, the solution is the use of an *ex post facto*, or *retrospective*, study. This term means that the difference between the two groups in relation to the independent variable has already happened and lies in the past (ex post facto means *'after the fact'*; Schmidt and Brown 2009). So, for instance, we might be interested in establishing whether going to antenatal classes has some impact on having a normal birth. It would be difficult to construct a study and allocate women to the antenatal class attendance group and others to the antenatal class non-attendance group, as it would mean withholding access to facilities to some people who might want to attend classes and for whom they would be beneficial.

An ex post facto study would collect data on women who had a normal birth and those that did not and try to establish if there was any pattern as to which group had the highest level of attendance at antenatal classes. In this design we are looking for associations provided by correlation. This statistical process allows us to identify the extent to which factors seem to go together. Unfortunately, we cannot say that one causes the other, only that they appear to be linked. However, this may be satisfactory in providing the basis for midwifery action, or increasing our ability to predict certain events.

The strength of both quasi-experimental and ex post facto designs is their practical nature. They are far more feasible and, because they avoid some of the ethical issues of experimental designs, are very attractive designs for midwifery research.

CONDUCTING RESEARCH

Experiments are not easy to carry out, so make sure it fits the research aim and then carefully follow the complex demands of this design. Where the purpose of your study is to establish a cause-and-effect relationship, an experimental approach is the method of choice. This will usually take the form of answering the question 'is approach/intervention A more effective than approach/intervention B'.

The key to planning an experimental design is to demonstrate the three defining elements of an experiment, namely:

- randomisation,
- manipulation,
- control.

Perhaps one of the most important parts of the design is how random allocation will be managed. This must be done systematically to ensure that everyone has an equal chance of being in the experiment or control group. A major part of the credibility of the study will rest on a convincing management of this aspect.

At an early stage, the researcher must consider the ethical issues raised by an experimental study, particularly in relation to possible harm through an intervention, or through withholding a known successful intervention. It is advisable to consult Chapter 8 on ethics to ensure that possible problem areas have been anticipated.

Previous research should be examined carefully, with special attention to design details. In particular, how did the researchers address the threats to internal and external validity? The literature should also provide clues as to the relevant independent variables to be included, and the additional variables that may confound the results, that is, cloud the ability to say that the results have been produced by the independent variable(s) manipulated in the study.

What is the hypothesis that will guide your study design? This should be a clear statement that includes the dependent and independent variable(s). Will the hypothesis be directional and predict that the results of the experimental group will be higher or lower than the control group (referred to as a *one-tailed hypothesis*), non-directional and suggest there will be a difference without saying whether it will be higher or lower in a particular group (referred to as a *two-tailed hypothesis*, as the results could go either way), or a *null-hypothesis*, where it states there would be no difference between the two groups (see Chapter 7)?

Thought should be given to what information will need to be collected to test the hypothesis. This will have to be in a numeric form, and will be subjected to a statistical test. There are a variety of tests, depending on the form of the experiment and the nature of the numeric values (see Chapter 13). It is at the early design stage that the necessary statistical procedures should be decided. It is recommended that help and advice is sought from someone who is knowledgeable in statistical techniques.

To reduce bias as much as possible, who will collect the data? In some instances it may be feasible, as well as highly desirable, to have someone not directly involved with the design of the study collect data 'blind', that is, without knowing whether subjects are in the experimental or control group. At the design stage, the necessity and method of blinding the subjects should be considered to produce a 'double-blind' study. Remember that in midwifery it is not always realistic to expect that those in the study will not know what intervention they have received.

Where several people are collecting data, steps should be taken to ensure they measure, code, or collect the information in exactly the same way and with the same degree of accuracy (referred to as *inter-rater* or *inter-observer reliability*). This attention to consistency and accuracy should extend to any equipment used as part of the study, or any materials such as Likert scales or other form of measurements.

The way the study is carried out must be carefully recorded in sufficient detail so that it can be replicated. A pilot study is essential to familiarise data collectors with the equipment and the procedure.

When conducting the main study, the safety and welfare of the subjects is paramount. This may lead to some individuals being removed from a study if there is any hint of personal danger.

At the end of an experimental study it is important to base the conclusions only on the statistically tested results. The statistical tests will indicate the strength of the relationship between the independent and dependent variables. However, there is always a margin of error in experimental studies. In addition, the sometimes artificial circumstances and environment of an experiment can make generalisations to practice difficult.

Where it is not possible, for practical or ethical reasons, to carry out a true experimental design, the next appropriate design such as quasi-experimental or ex post facto designs may be used. The rigour is just as important in these designs as in experimental designs, if not more so. This is because they will be viewed as weaker than an experimental design. Clear attempts should therefore be made to reduce the possibility of the results being explained by factors other than the ones being suggested by the researcher.

All the designs in this section depend on a very clear statistical presentation of the results. It is this aspect of research reports that many midwives can find most demanding. For this reason, the midwifery researcher should explain the statistical procedures used, and clarify their meaning and implications for the reader as simply as possible.

CRITIQUING RESEARCH

Critiquing experimental research can be challenging, often because of the reader's unfamiliarity with statistical presentation. Yet a little knowledge and understanding of some of the basic concepts and conventions can clarify the report drastically (see Chapter 13). The first stage of critiquing is to ensure that the researcher is searching for a cause-and-effect relationship between an independent and a dependent variable. This will usually be evident from the wording of the aim that will suggest the influence of one variable on another. Usually it will try to answer the question whether one treatment or action is 'more effective' than an alternative. Experimental research should contain a hypothesis, although, sadly, this is not present in all reports.

In examining the details of the conduct of the study, the three features of an experiment, *randomisation, manipulation*, and *control*, should be present. If randomisation or control is not present, it may be a quasi-experimental study. Often, the study will state this.

Where the study is clearly experimental, consideration should be given to the ethical component. Was the study approved by an ethics committee or, in the case of an American article, an institutional review board (IRB)? To what extent did those in the study clearly give their informed consent and has the avoidance of harm been addressed?

The sample included in the study should be scrutinised in relation to the inclusion and exclusion criteria for those selected for the study. Those in the sample should be typical of those in the larger group they represent. The method of randomisation should be examined to ensure that everyone had an equal chance of being selected for the experimental group. There will often be a diagram showing the flow of people into the different parts, or 'arms', of the study and showing how many entered or left the study at different points. This allows you to follow the numbers involved right down to the start of the study and perhaps through to the end of the study period. A close comparison should then be made of those in the final groups to ensure that they are comparable in those factors that might have made a difference to the results. Remember, they should be as similar as possible in all respects apart from the exposure to the independent variable under investigation.

The researcher should give clear concept and operational definitions for the dependent and independent variables. These definitions should be considered for their adequacy. The intervention should be provided in a standardised way to everyone. Was there a check on this, such as training for those involved in providing the intervention, to ensure consistency? In particular, an assessment should be made of possible inaccuracies in the measurements made following the intervention. Have the issues of reliability and validity been addressed to your satisfaction? In particular, have they measured what they think has been measured (validity)? Was this a blind or double-blind study? Are details provided of how these were achieved? If there was no blinding, could this have had an effect on the results?

In the results section, has the researcher used a test of significance to test the probability that any differences between groups could have happened by chance? Here, the size of the 'p' value is important. To what extent has the researcher taken into account the possible threats to internal and external validity? It is worth considering whether the results could be explained by some other factor besides the independent variable.

Depending on the results, what are the implications for practice? What specific recommendations are made in the report? Finally, are you satisfied with the rigour with which the researcher conducted the study? Is there a striving for excellence in the way the whole study was designed and carried out?

Above all, do not simply be impressed by the size of the study, its complexity, or the use of statistics. As with any kind of study, it is crucial to challenge the research. Consider the researcher's attempts to maintain accuracy and avoid bias and the limitations of their study. These will have implications for the extent to which you can generalise the results to your own clinical setting. With all clinical trials, it is wise to look for confirmation from replication studies before adopting a system that may have considerable implications for individual safety and quality of care.

KEY POINTS

- Experimental designs, particularly in the form of the randomised control trial, have become one of the most respected types of research in evidence-based practice. The reason for this relates to the way that drugs and treatments in the past have been carefully tested to reduce the possibility of other explanations for the results.
- The way experimental studies are carried out can be very complex because they are dependent on the three necessary experimental elements of randomisation, control, and manipulation. In midwifery, it is not always possible, or desirable, to achieve these elements. Sometimes it would be unethical, or would drastically reduce women's choice or individual midwife's judgement as to what was best in the particular circumstances, if strict experimental protocols were followed.

- There are alternatives to a full experimental design, such as quasi-experimental, ex post facto and correlation designs. Although these do not produce conclusions that are as 'strong' as experimental designs, they can still inform evidence-based practice.
- Despite the status given to experimental designs, they do have limitations. It is not always possible to control for other factors that might explain the results. In addition, it is sometimes an oversimplification to look for one cause for a phenomenon; sometimes there are several.
- The power of this type of design depends on the use of statistical methods, particularly inferential statistics. These identify the role of chance in explaining the difference in the results between groups. The knowledge required to understand this form of research is more demanding than in other methods. However, midwives should not see this as a reason for avoiding experimental approaches, or avoid reading published experimental studies. The effort needed to gain the statistical knowledge and understanding is well worth the reward of being able to confidently use and challenge this research approach.

REFERENCES

Burns, N., Grove, S., 2009. The Practice of Nursing Research: Appraisal, Synthesis, and Generation of Evidence. sixth ed. Saunders, St Louis.

Cambell, D., Stanley, J., 1963. Experimental and Quasi-experimental Design. Rand McNally, Chicago.

McDonald, S., Henderson, J., Faulkner, S., Evans, S., Hagan, R., 2010. Effect of an extended midwifery postnatal support programme on the duration of breast feeding: A randomised controlled trial. Midwifery 26 (1), 88–100.

Nelson, A., Dumville, J., Torgerson, D., 2010. Experimental research. In: Gerrish, K., Lacey, A. (Eds.), The Research Process in Nursing. sixth ed. Wiley-Blackwell, Chichester.

Norman, I., Humphrey, C., 2008. Evaluation research. In: Watson, R., McKenna, H., Cowman, S., Keady, J. (Eds.), Nursing Research: Designs and Methods. Edinburgh, Churchill Livingstone.

O'Sullivan, G., Liu, B., Hart, D., Seed, P., Shennan, A., 2009. Effect of food intake during labour on obstetric outcome: randomised controlled trial. Br. Med. J. Online: doi:10.1136/bmj.b784.

Polit, D., Beck, C., 2008. Nursing Research: Generating and Assessing Evidence for Nursing Practice. eighth ed. Lippincott Williams and Wilkins, Philadelphia.

Schmidt, N., Brown, J., 2009. Evidence-Based Practice for Nurses: Appraisal and Application of Research. Jones and Bartlett, Sudbury.

Smith, G., 2008. Experiments. In: Watson, R., McKenna, H., Cowman, S., Keady, J. (Eds.), Nursing Research: Designs and Methods. Edinburgh, Churchill Livingstone.

Spiby, H., Munro, J. (Eds.), 2010. Evidence Based Midwifery: Applications in Context. Wiley-Blackwell, Chichester.

Svensson, J., Barclay, L., Cooke, M., 2009. Randomised-controlled trial of two antenatal education programmes. Midwifery 25 (2), 114–125.

Wallace, L., Dunn, O., Alder, E., Inch, S., Hills, R., Law, S., 2006. A randomised-controlled trial in England of a postnatal midwifery intervention on breast-feeding duration. Midwifery 22 (3), 262–273.

Wood, M., Ross-Kerr, J., 2006. Basic Steps in Planning Nursing Research: From question to Proposal. sixth ed. Jones and Bartlett, Boston.

Statistics in research

13

This is the chapter you may be tempted to skip; however, do not pass on just yet. Understanding the way numbers are presented in research is one of the most important skills that will help you in making sense of research articles. It is also an essential chapter if you have to present your own quantitative findings in research or audit. To read research papers in greater depth, every midwife needs to understand some of the key statistical principles that will help in deciding in quantitative research whether the author's conclusions are justified. So, although it is easy to ignore the statistical sections in research, understanding them can have a direct effect on care. Indeed, Spiby and Munro (2010) suggest that if midwives are to integrate evidence-based practice into their care, they must understand research and be able to interpret the data on which it is based.

The aim of this chapter is to explain just some of the common statistical ideas used in quantitative research, the basic principles underpinning them, and how to interpret them.

COMMON ATTITUDES TO STATISTICS

Once quantitative researchers have gathered the data from their study, they are faced with transforming the raw results into some kind of order that can be understood. Any summary and presentation of the data will involve numbers and statistical processes and this is where the problems can start. For many people, the way numbers are presented and the statistical techniques applied to the data creates problems, and is the point at which some readers decide either to ignore the numbers, or put down the article.

Why do statistics make so many people turn cold? Perhaps they remind us of unpleasant experiences in school where we felt lost or left behind. For some, the easiest way of coping with these feelings is to give up, and pretend statistics do not matter. Unfortunately, they do. For those ready to make a fresh start, this chapter will explain just a small selection of some of the statistical procedures you will meet in many research reports. You will not have to learn how to carry out complicated calculations; there are specialised books and courses that will help you if you need to know this. For those carrying out research there are also people with this expertise to draw on, but you do have to know what to ask.

If the very word 'statistics' frightens you, let us start by acknowledging that without statistics the results of any study would just be a chaotic jumble of numbers that would provide little meaning (Polit and Beck 2008). Statistical processes bring order and understanding to all the information that has been collected.

As with research in general, there are some unusual words and symbols to learn and some familiar words that have different meanings (see Table 13.1). One example is the word *'significant'*. This does not mean 'important', but suggests that the difference in the outcomes between two groups in, say, a randomised control trial (RCT), is unlikely to have happened by chance. In other words, the difference between the two groups is more likely to be explained by what the researcher did than by any other explanation. For this reason, when talking or writing about research, unless you are using it in its statistical sense, it is better to avoid saying something is 'significant'. Similarly, the word *'data'* is plural, so you will see the word *'are'* not *'is'* following it, as well as expressions such as 'the data *were* calculated', not *'was'* calculated.

Finally, at the start of this chapter we should dismiss a common misconception about statistics. It is not true to say *'you can prove anything with statistics'* – rather, some people can misuse them or ignore the rules that affect their use. This is where the reader must have some understanding of statistics in order to suspect that the results do not support the conclusions being made. However, most research papers are based on a relatively small number of accepted procedures and assumptions. You do not have to understand exactly how something was calculated, as long as you understand the basic principles underpinning its use and you can 'read' the symbols and statements used by the researcher.

A SIMPLE DIFFERENCE

There are two major categories of statistic used in research: *descriptive* statistics and *inferential* statistics. Descriptive statistics use numbers to paint a picture of features or variables found in a sample, whilst inferential statistics are used to apply the findings from the sample to the wider population from which it was taken, or to test the truth of a hypothesis. Inferential statistics are an essential part of RCTs as they indicate the extent to which the intervention introduced by the researcher had an impact on the outcome. Inferential statistics also include the use of *correlation*; this indicates a pattern or association between variables, for example, in a survey. Each of these two categories of statistic will now be examined.

DESCRIPTIVE STATISTICS

Quantitative research is concerned with measuring a variable in a way that produces a numeric value. Some variables such as weight, time, and amount of fluid lost have clear operational definitions in the form of standard units of

Table 13.1 Common statistical symbols and their meaning

Symbol	Meaning	Use
Σ	Greek symbol meaning add together what follows	As part of a formula providing instructions, e.g. Σx, which means add together each value for the variable collected.
<	Less than	Indicates set value e.g. $P < 0.05$ means that the value of P is below or smaller than 0.05.
>	Greater than	Indicates the opposite of the above as in $P > 0.05$, which means that the value is greater than 0.05. The open end of the symbol means greater than, and the closed end means less than reading from the left hand side of the symbol.
$\geq$	Equal to or greater than	To indicate a condition to be met during a calculation.
$\pm$	Plus and minus the figure that follows	Used for example in standard deviation (sd) where the figure that follows the symbol is taken away from the mean and then added to the mean to give the range between which the majority of values in the data set will fall.
χ^2	Symbol for the chi-squared test (pronounced 'ki-squared') as in kite	This test indicates the chances that any differences between the groups in the study could have happened by chance. The test is used with 'nominal data' (i.e. falling into one category or another, such as yes or no) and compares the actual results with what might have been expected if there was no difference between the groups.
$p < 0.05$	Used as part of statistical tests to indicate the level of probability of being wrong if a real difference between the groups involved was assumed	This is the minimum level set for tests of significance to indicate that the results are unlikely to have happened purely by chance. Roughly, it means you would be wrong 5 times in 100 if you said there was a real difference between the groups involved. Other values showing a progressively better result include $p < 0.01$ (1 in 100), and $p < 0.001$ (1 in a 1000).
NS	Non-significant	This abbreviation suggests that there was not a statistical difference between the outcomes of an experimental and control group. Testing has failed to reach the level $p < 0.05$; therefore the study has failed to demonstrate a real difference between the groups concerned.
r_s	The symbol for Spearman's rho (pronounced 'row')	Used to indicate a correlation between two variables measured at least at ordinal level. The strength of this will be somewhere between $+1$ and -1.
r	The symbol for the Pearson Product-moment (usually referred to as Pearson r)	The same as the above only this is used where both variables are measured at either interval or ratio level. This falls into the category of parametric statistics as it indicates features (parameters) of the population from which the sample is taken.

(Continued)

Table 13.1 Common statistical symbols and their meaning—cont'd

Symbol	Meaning	Use
t	The *t*-test symbol	This parametric test examines the difference in the means of two groups to see if they are statistically different. There are two versions, the *t*-test for independent samples, i.e. two different groups, and the *t*-test for matched or paired groups, i.e. the same group before and after an intervention.
CI	Confidence Interval	This is an upper and lower figure between which the value measured in the sample is estimated to lie in the population as a whole.

measurement, such as kilograms, minutes and millilitres. For some attributes, such as the physical condition of a baby at birth, scales have been devised in the form of an Apgar score. Other elements such as satisfaction with the birth, or the amount of information received on screening procedures, may have to be turned into numeric values. This is achieved using approximate measures such as Likert scales, where individuals answer a number of statements using options such as 'strongly agree', 'agree'. The researcher then gives each choice a number, such as:

Strongly agree	Agree	Undecided	Disagree	Strongly disagree
5	4	3	2	1

The basic principle behind all these procedures is to provide the researcher with some form of numeric measurement that can be processed statistically.

From these examples, it can be seen that some numbers express quantities that are more precise and exact, while others are a more general statement of quantity. Time and volume can be checked and agreed objectively as accurate. Other measurements are less precise and objective, for example, an estimation of blood loss or dilatation of the cervix. This is an important observation, as some researchers will claim a greater degree of objectivity and accuracy for their data than is possible. For some studies, numbers have been produced more as a convenience to allow statistical procedures to take place than as a precise measurement.

LEVELS OF MEASUREMENT

All numbers look the same. It is possible to construct any combination of numbers you like using the numbers 0 to 9. In statistical theory, numbers are used to represent different ideas, depending on the characteristics of the number. One simple but very important categorisation is the following four *levels of measurement*:

1. Nominal level (or categorical level)

This is the most basic level. It places or 'nominates' a variable into a particular category that is mutually exclusive (it can only be put into one category) and uses a number as a label for that category. So midwives working only in the community may be categorised under the heading '1', and midwives working only in the hospital setting could be categorised as '2', those working in both might be '3'. This means that those in the category '1' are the same or equivalent; it does not mean that it takes two community midwives to make one hospital midwife; it just provides a label that happens to be a number, it is not a measurement of quantity. They could just as easily have been labelled using a letter of the alphabet, as in the case of blood groups, a colour or anything else.

2. Ordinal level

As we go up each level, the higher category has the characteristics of the level below, but has extra, more advanced, qualities. So, numbers in this second group not only label a category but also indicate sequence or rank order. For example, arrivals at a clinical area might be given the sequential numeric values 1, 2, 3, 4 to indicate the order in which they entered that area. This would indicate that number 3 was two behind number 1, and one ahead of number 4. However, we cannot do much more with the numbers. We do not know how much later each person was behind the one in front. There may have been a split second between numbers 1 and 2 and several hours before number 3 entered and a day before number 4 entered.

The relevance of this category of measurement is that it takes the same form of the numbers used in a Likert scale or Apgar score. Although the parts of the scale can be labelled 1 to 5, as in the case of a Likert scale, there is no indication of the precise distance between each point. The distance between 'agree' and 'strongly agree', may not be the same as that between 'disagree' and 'strongly disagree'. All that we can say is that the numbers indicate sequence or rank order along a continuum.

Both nominal and ordinal levels of measurement form a single subcategory in the levels of measurement called *categorical data* – they put things in categories that are identified by a number, and do not measured quantitatively. They both possess very basic properties that restrict the statistical procedures that can be carried out on them. The next two categories are far more sophisticated and provide more useful information.

3. Interval level

This level produces numbers that allocate units to a category, indicate sequence, but this time the distances between the different points are the same. This means that they can be 'averaged', and have other procedures carried out on them. Along with the next category, the interval level indicates 'true numbers' that measures amounts, and does not simply use numbers as a label.

4. Ratio level

This is the final, and highest, level of measurement. It is very much like the interval level except for one crucial factor, and that is there is an absolute zero point in the measurement scale below which it is impossible to record a value. For example, temperature readings in Fahrenheit or centigrade are interval level because it is possible to have a minus figure, such as minus five degrees centigrade. This is because zero in Fahrenheit and centigrade are arbitrary points, not an absolute zero. Height, age and weight are all ratio level as it is impossible to have less than a zero amount of any of them.

The importance of the last two levels of measurement is that they quantify something, and they are always measured in units of some kind, such as kilograms, hours and minutes, centilitres. It is this property that makes them suitable for statistical procedures in that the other levels of nominal and ordinal do not measure the quantity of anything but simply categorise, using numbers to label the categories, and in the case of ordinal data, place them in sequence. For this reason, the interval and ratio levels are classed as numeric levels and the nominal and ordinal levels are seen as categorical levels. The key characteristics of these four levels of measurement are summarised in Table 13.2.

Space has been devoted to the explanation of these levels as many of the principles of statistical analysis are based on this categorisation system; therefore, their importance to understanding statistics should not be underestimated. In the next section we turn to the problem of making descriptive statistics meaningful to the reader.

SUMMARISING DESCRIPTIVE DATA: MEASURES OF CENTRAL TENDENCY

Burns and Grove (2009) point out that although analysing the results of a study is one of the most exciting parts of a study for the researcher, this can be one of the most challenging aspects for the reader of a research report. Yet the reason for processing data is to make them easier to understand. It is no use presenting results in terms of each person's answers to a questionnaire or physical assessment expressed in the numeric values for each answer, as in the following:

| Respondent A: | 21 | 2 | 29 | 17 | 2 | 55 | 34 | 23 | 7 | 81 | 64 | 34 | 3 | 29 | 46 | 50 |
| Respondent B: | 18 | 37 | 4 | 21 | 31 | 8 | 30 | 15 | 1 | 2 | 57 | 41 | 75 | 4 | 7 | 47 |

It would mean very little as it is not clear to what the numbers relate, and there is no pattern visible that makes sense between the two respondents. The answer is to use summary statistics that allow us to convey meaning by summarising quite large collections of numbers.

Table 13.2 *Properties and characteristics of each level of measurement*

Level	Properties	Characteristics
Nominal	Most basic of all	Names, categorises variables
Ordinal	Basic non-measurement	Numbers used to categorise into sequence or 'rank order'
Interval	Measures properties of variable	Equal distance between units; no absolute zero. Sophisticated statistical procedures possible
Ratio	Highest level	Absolute zero, equal distance between units. Suited to sophisticated statistical procedures

The most successful form of summary statistic is the *measure of central tendency*. This is a clumsy way of saying the number that appears typical in the group, or the number that represents the central value found in the entire collection of results (data set). If you are thinking 'that sounds like the average' you would be right, but in statistics there are a number of different ways of calculating 'the average', each known by a different name.

1. Mean

This is what we commonly call the 'average'. For instance, we might say 'on average, I take half an hour to get home from work', or we might read that 'on average, people watch television for four hours a day'. We don't mean that the figure is exact; sometimes it may be more, sometimes in may be less, but when we even things out it is reasonably typical.

It is not difficult to calculate the 'average' or 'mean' of something. If you had to work out the average length of time that 10 members of staff in your clinical area had been qualified, you would ask each one how long they had been qualified, add them all together and divide by the total number of people. Easy! To write down that process so others could repeat it, the statistician would symbolise each stage to produce the following formula:

$$\frac{\Sigma X}{N}$$

The symbols translate as:
Σ = Add together each of the following
X = The numeric value of the item you are interested in from each person
— = The sign for 'divide by' used in a fraction
N = The total number in the group.

The formula looks baffling, but understanding the symbols, and the sequence in which to carry out the procedures, makes it clearer. This is how even the most complicated formulae work; each symbol is translated into an instruction that is carried out in a set sequence.

The mean can only be calculated if the level of data is either interval or ratio, that is, where the numbers reach a numeric level of measurement and are actually measuring something in recognisable units of quantity. It does not work for categorical data such as calculating the average star sign of people in a group where Aquarius = 1, Pisces = 2, etc. Neither does it really work with ordinal data, although you will see an average figure for Likert scale values calculated.

There is one big drawback in using the mean, and that is it is influenced by untypical numbers that are much higher or much lower than the majority of other numbers in the group or 'data set'. These more extreme values are called *'outliers'*, because when individual results are plotted on a graph, they are the ones that stand out because they are out of line with the main results. The result would be an untypical value of what is typical in the group and so we can sometimes be misled by the mean for a group of results because there may be a small number of untypical results pulling the mean up or down. This is illustrated in Box 13.1.

> **BOX 13.1 Ages of those attending a restaurant party**
>
> a) Ages of a group of children going to a birthday party
>   6 6 8 8 9 9 10 11 11
>   median = 9, mean = 8.6
> b) Ages of children plus Grandma and her twin sister Elsie going to a birthday party
>   6 6 8 8 9 9 10 72 72
>   median = 9, mean = 22.2
>
> **Punch line**: The median is a more stable calculation, as outliers (untypical large or small figures) do not influence it; the mean is influenced by outliers and can produce an unrepresentative figure.

2. Median

The median is a useful calculation of central tendency, as it is not influenced by extreme values. The median is calculated by taking every single figure in the set of numbers, such as length of second stage of labour for 20 women. They are all then put in rank order from the smallest to the biggest. The median is the value of the unit in the middle of this row or *distribution* of numbers.

Let us take an example to illustrate the advantage of the median over the mean. Imagine nine children have been booked for a birthday party at a restaurant. Unfortunately, the only information the restaurant has to prepare for the type of party is the name of the person who made the booking. They need to know whether to provide a children's jelly and blancmange type party, or a fairly wild alcoholic affair. The solution is to telephone and ask for the average (mean) age of those attending.

If the set of ages (values) in line a) in Box 13.1 were used to supply the mean, the figure communicated would be 8.6 or, corrected up to the nearest whole figure, 9 years. The median could be calculated once each item in the data set had been put in rank order from the smallest to the biggest (which has already been done), by identifying the 'middle' value. This would be the fifth number, as there would be four numbers on either side of it. In this example, the median would also be 9 years.

Now what if the two 11-year-olds felt they were too old for such a 'childish' celebration and decided to back out, leaving Grandma and her twin sister Elsie, both 72, to accompany the children instead? If the restaurant rang up this time to be told the average age in the party was 22.2, or 22 to the nearest whole figure, they may lay on a very alcoholic adult type of birthday party. However, if they had asked for the median, the value would have still been 9, because it is the position in the rank order that is used to calculate the answer, not the combined values.

How is the median calculated where there is an even number of items in the data set, as in the set below?

6 6 8 8 9 9 10 11

The answer is to first identify the midpoint again. This time it would be a line drawn between 8 and 9, as there would be 4 values on each side of the line. Simply adding the values of the numbers either side of the line together and dividing by two would produce the median of 8.5 (8+9 = 17÷2 = 8.5) years. In other words, it is the mean of the combined values of the numbers on either side of the line that splits the ranked sequence of numbers into two halves.

A good way of remembering what is achieved through calculating the median is that it provides a cut-off point along a ranked order of numbers so that half of all the values are below that cut-off point; the median value, and the remaining half are above it.

There is one disadvantage of the median, and that is it becomes very unwieldy to calculate if there is a very large set of values in the data set, as each one has to be placed in rank order to locate the middle value. However, knowing both the mean and the median will give you an insight into whether there are outliers in the distribution. The closer the two values are together, the less likely there is to be outliers affecting the mean.

3. Mode

The final method of calculating an average is the mode. This is the most frequently appearing value in the data set. If we go back to the set of values in b) in Box 13.1 above, and adjust it slightly to make it:

c) Adjusted distribution of ages

6 6 6 8 8 9 9 10 72 72

The mode would be 6, as that is the number that appears the greatest number of times. However, if there were three 6-year-olds and three 9-year-olds, then there would be two modes, 6 and 9. This is referred to as a *bimodal distribution*. Just to complicate things, if there had been three 8-year-olds as well as three 6-year-olds and three 9-year-olds, it would have been *multimodal*.

You are probably already getting the feeling that this is not a very useful way of saying what is typical in the group, as the mode can change drastically as a result of one number that can shift the mode anywhere in the distribution. This can be confirmed by taking c) above and changing the first and last digit as follows:

d) Final adjustment of ages

6 6 8 8 9 9 10 72 72 72

We have now swung the mode from one end of the line to the other end by just changing two numbers. This illustrates the point that each statistical calculation has its own special characteristics, and we have to know something about these in order to know when they can be misleading. When painting a picture of what is typical in a group of results (or data set), or what is around the middle value, we have to be very careful which method of calculation we choose, as we can alter the result radically by using a different calculation.

MEASURES OF CENTRAL TENDENCY: THE STANDARD DEVIATION

The last section illustrated that the mean is not the most useful method of calculating the value that stands for, or is typical of, the values in the group. The final statistical method in this section allows us to go back to the mean and make it more useful by using the mean in combination with the *standard deviation*.

The standard deviation (abbreviated to 'sd') is a measurement derived by working out the average distance of each item in a data set from the mean. If we measured 30 women's heights, the mean might be 1.62 metres. The standard deviation, when calculated to establish the mean distance of each woman's height from the overall mean, might work out at 8 cm. The value of the standard deviation is then added to the mean (1.62 m + 8 cm) to give 1.70 m as an upper value, and is then taken away from the mean (1.62 m − 8 cm) to give 1.54 m as a lower value. Where there is an even pattern in the variable concerned (explained in the following section under the heading 'normal distribution'), the majority of people (around 68%) will lie in this range between the mean and plus and minus one standard deviation (±1sd).

The smaller the standard deviation in relation to the mean, the closer all the values will be to the mean. This would suggest that the mean is reasonably typical of the values in the group. The larger the standard deviation, the more spread out the values will be, as there will be a large variation between the values above and below the mean (the mean plus and minus the standard deviation). In this case, this indicates that the mean is not very helpful in gaining an idea of what is typical in the group.

The standard deviation is also used to identify if the attributes of those in two groups, for example in an RCT, are closely matched, or whether they are different, and if so, how different. This is achieved by comparing the mean and standard deviation in the two groups. We would not expect the results to be identical, but we would want to feel they were reasonably close and that any discrepancies did not suggest clinically significant variations that might make a difference to the interpretation of the results.

NORMAL DISTRIBUTION

In looking at the way individual values are spread around the mean, there is one particular pattern they can take that is important to the statistician, and this is called the *normal distribution*. Normal distribution is a theoretical concept that has a major influence on a number of important statistical decisions, including those in inferential statistics, discussed below. It relates to interval and ratio data and can be outlined as follows. If we were to plot the frequency distribution of characteristics such as height or blood pressure from a large number of people on a graph, they would form a very distinctive shape. This is because in a large sample the numbers of very tall people and the numbers of very short people appear in about the same ratio with the majority of people being fairly close to the mean height. The curve on the graph would look like the outline of a church bell, where the majority of people would be in the mid section and the slope of the curve of the bell shape would come down to the small number of people, on either side of the majority, who were either very tall or very short (see Figure 13.1).

The distinctive characteristic of such distribution is that the mean, mode and median would all hit the same value. This would appear on a graph as one line passing from the very apex of the bell (the tallest point on the curve)

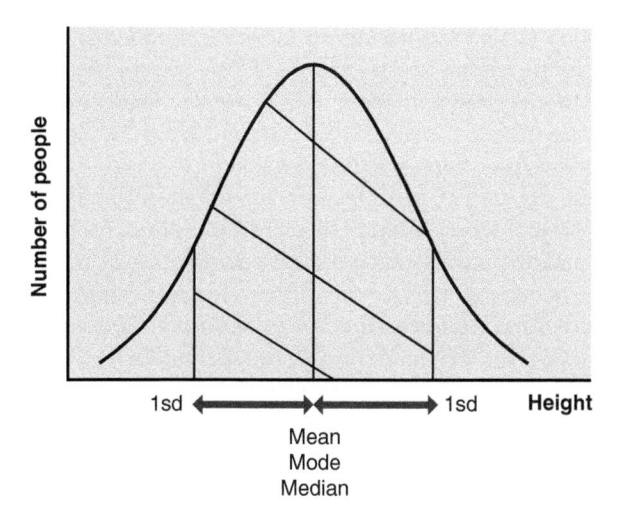

FIG 13.1 Normal distribution curve showing the height of a group of people.

to the baseline of the graph. The shape is said to be symmetrical, in that if we were to cut the shape out of the page on which it appeared, and fold it down the midline formed by the mean, each side would touch perfectly like a mirror image, without any overlaps.

This kind of a shape has a mathematical property whereby if we measure one standard deviation either side of this midline, then the area under the curve inside the lines formed by the upper and lower standard deviation points would include the values from about 68% of all the individuals in the study. This is a constant result for all variables that have a normal distribution.

The usefulness of this is that if a variable is reasonably normally distributed and we know the mean, by calculating the standard deviation and working out one standard deviation above and below the mean, we can be sure that the majority of people in the sample (68%) will measure somewhere between this upper and lower level of measurement. This can be extended to two standard deviations ($\pm 2\,sd$) to give an upper and lower level between which about 95% of all the values will fall. However, most studies use one standard deviation to give a picture of the majority of measurements.

It is worth ending by saying that this idea of a normal distribution is part of statistical theory, and as Burns and Grove (2009) point out, distributions in reality will rarely exactly fit the normal distribution. Nevertheless, it is taken as providing a reasonably useful guide to producing meaningful statistical interpretations of results.

PRESENTATION OF DESCRIPTIVE RESULTS

Having looked at some of the basic principles of descriptive statistics, we can look at common diagrammatical ways of presenting results, and how we can make sense of them. Although researchers will describe the results in words in the main body or text of their report, they will frequently use some visual displays to help the reader 'see' the results. This visual presentation can take a number of forms, as shown in Table 13.3. These can include summary tables, which present the major numerical findings, and graphical figures such as bar charts, histograms, pie charts and line graphs.

Each of these can convey complex information more efficiently than words because of the visual representation of a large amount of numbers. An examination of a visual display also allows the reader to observe the overall pattern or trend of the results, which is more difficult to understand when presented in the form of words. However, the researcher must choose the right format for the information, and the reader must understand the principles and shorthand used by the writer. Any form of visual display must also be presented in such a way that they do not mislead the reader in interpreting the results (Walters and Freeman 2010).

Although Table 13.3 outlines a range of common data presentation forms, for many people reading research reports, the tables, charts and diagrams can become like holes in the page; they don't really exist. This is because we do not teach people how to read tables and diagrams. The next section is an attempt to overcome this with the help of some guidelines.

How to read tables?

Tables, according to Atkinson (2008), form the most popular choice for presenting numeric data in research as they allow the results of a variety of variables to be presented side by side to give a clear overview. In this way, the

Table 13.3 *Common methods of presenting descriptive data*

Type	Description
Tables	Labelled columns and rows of numbers. Can take the form of frequency tables, where just one variable is examined, or cross-tabulations where two or more variables are shown. One variable can then be displayed in terms of another variable (intention to breast feed or bottle feed by parity).
Bar charts	A block diagram used to show amounts of a discrete (cannot be broken down into smaller units) variable, such as male/female. The blocks, or 'bars', do not touch. They can be shown in a vertical format or horizontal format. They can be 'stacked' bar charts, where each bar totals 100% and is divided within its length into sub groups by proportion.
Histograms	As above, but shows a continuous (can be broken down into smaller units of measurement) variable. The blocks will touch to show they are on a continuous scale.
Pie charts	This is a circle divided into appropriate 'slices' to show the quantity of different categories. The result must add up to 100%. These work well when there are between three and six slices providing the majority of slices are not too 'thin'.
Line graph	Lines that join points plotted on a graph to show trends in the data.

purpose of a table is to create a kind of numeric photograph of a situation in long shot, but at the same time allow the reader to zoom in to close-up by examining particular squares, or 'cells', in the table.

Tables come in two different kinds: a *frequency table* and a *cross-tabulation* or *contingency table*. A frequency table looks at how often (frequently) categories of one variable occurred in the data. For example, Table 13.4 illustrates a frequency table for age of a sample of women in a survey.

The second type of table takes the frequency table, and looks for possible patterns by introducing another variable, such as parity, so that the first variable is broken down into another variable. This is called a *cross-tabulation* or *contingency table*, where one factor is 'contingent', that is, conditional or dependent, on another. An illustration of this type of table is shown in Table 13.5 where parity is cross-tabulated with age in a second survey of women.

Table 13.4 *Example of a frequency table: age distribution of sample*

Age group	Number	(%)
< 18	23	10.3
18–21	47	21.2
22–26	53	23.9
27–30	42	18.9
31–34	35	15.8
35+	22	9.9
Total	222	100.0

Table 13.5 *Example of a cross-tabulation: parity of study sample by age group*

Age group	Primagravida Number	(%)	Multigravida Number	(%)
< 18	32	(17.5)	2	(1.0)
18–21	40	(21.9)	31	(15.3)
22–26	42	(23.0)	47	(23.1)
27–30	34	(18.5)	54	(26.6)
31–34	23	(12.6)	40	(19.7)
35+	12	(6.5)	29	(14.3)
Total	183	(100.0)	203	(100.0)

When reading a table, the first task is to examine the layout and headings. You might want to read the following and look at a cross-tabulation from an article at the same time. Start by establishing from the title what the table represents. Is there just one variable, which would indicate a frequency table, or is it a cross-tabulation with two or more variables? This will help you anticipate what kind of a pattern it may contain. Then look at the columns and rows. Each should be clearly labelled at the top of the columns, and to the left of the rows. This helps you to 'read' the table in terms of what the numbers 'stand for' or represent.

A useful starting point for exploring a summary table is to look down each column for the highest numbers to get a feel for which item or category was the largest. Ask yourself, 'Is that what I would have expected?' How close in value are the other items to the highest? Again, is that what you could have expected, or is this an unexpected, clinically relevant finding? You can also consider the reverse of this by identifying which categories have the smallest values. Could you have anticipated that or is it unusual? Look too at the relative size or pattern in the values of all the numbers. This will give you some idea of the rank order of the items in terms of which is the highest, the next highest, and so on. Some tables may present the order of the rows in rank order as part of the format. Do these numbers go down gradually in size, or are there some items with large values followed by a sudden drop down to the next value? This will tell you if there is some consistency in the distribution, or whether most responses fell into a small number of categories that were mentioned by, or typical of, most people in the study.

Where there are a number of columns in the table, it is useful to make comparisons across each item indicated by the row headings to see if the value of the number in each column is similar or different. If different, are the differences small or large? As you start to identify patterns amongst the results, ask yourself the following questions:

- What does this suggest to me?
- Is this what I would expect or not?
- So what?

This type of reflection and analysis will provide you with opinions about the findings and how they relate to the study aim. What could be the 'story' or explanation behind the findings? Your answers can then be compared with the researcher's comments on each table. Examine the tables before you read the researcher's comments, so that you do not simply accept what is said unquestioningly.

These points are also useful if you need to construct tables. The first point is to establish if the information will be easier to communicate in the form of a summary table. If the answer is 'yes', then you will need to identify how much information you need to put in each table. Avoid overloading the reader with too much information. However, sometimes it is easier to compare two situations, such as Caesarean section rate between primigravida and multigravida women by putting them in the same table to make comparisons and contrasts more evident.

Tables from randomised control trials (RCTs)

Where the table represents the results from an RCT, there are certain conventions the researcher should observe. These include which variables are shown as columns or rows. The convention is that column headings are used to display the independent variable and the row headings indicate the dependent variable. The purpose is to allow the researcher to see any patterns in the data.

To help you answer the question of what the table shows, the researcher will indicate if they have used inferential statistics on the table, and what was found. This is indicated either underneath the table or as a column in the table, where the researcher should indicate the statistical test used, the result, and the 'p' value, which indicates whether the differences could have happened purely by chance (see Chapter 12).

Making sense of bar charts and pie charts

Although tables provide an overall view of data, and allow us to zoom in on specific parts, we have to interpret and keep track of a lot of ideas in our head. This means we have to visualise differences in size between quantities. Bar charts, histograms and pie charts are different, as they provide instant visual comparisons. However, we still have to know something of the conventions surrounding such displays, so that we can read them easily.

Bar charts contain a series of rectangles or 'blocks' presented either vertically or horizontally, and represent the values or scores for a number of categories. They are an ideal way of highlighting comparisons between variables. This can be between two or more variables where the height or length of the bars will draw attention to differences between them. Good bar charts are presented in size order from the largest down to the smallest. This helps the eye and brain follow the relative differences in size easier.

Histograms are similar in appearance to bar charts, but each block touches those on either side of them as the data they represent are on a continuous scale ranging from zero upwards. In most bar charts, the order of the blocks does not matter, as they are separate (discrete) items and could be reordered without changing the meaning, for example reasons given for giving up breastfeeding (McDonald et al. 2010). These are separate categories and could be moved around depending on the numbers choosing each category. In histograms, this would be impossible, as with variables such as height, weight, or number of weeks' breastfeeding, the order of the blocks cannot be rearranged without destroying the natural sequence.

Making sense of bar charts, and histograms, is a matter of comparison between blocks and establishing the overall pattern on display. The essential question to answer is: 'How does this relate to the research aim?' Is the pattern important to the research, and is it clinically relevant? In examining such charts, look carefully at the size of the scale used, as the author or publishers can make a small difference between two outcomes seem quite large, merely by making the scale of the diagram bigger. It is always wise, therefore, to consider the question: 'Is the difference really remarkable, or does the scale of the figure exaggerate the relative differences?'

Pie charts are another common form of graphic presentation of results. A pie chart is a circle 'sliced-up' to represent the relative proportion of each of the categories in a response. Pie charts work well with nominal or categorical levels of measurement, where all the items added together make up a total of 100% (so people cannot chose or fall into more than one category). Although these are really helpful to compare one variable in proportion to another as part of the whole, they do not work well once the number of 'slices' exceeds five (Walters and Freeman 2010).

All the data presentation methods described in this section serve the same purpose, that is, to convey the results of data analysis quickly, clearly and meaningfully. The problem for the researcher is to show the results in a way that will be easily assimilated by the reader, and will make the interpretation of the data clear and interesting. When reading research reports, all forms of presenting the data should be carefully examined and not overlooked; remember, 'every picture tells a story'.

INFERENTIAL STATISTICS

So far, we have considered descriptive statistics in depth, and mentioned inferential statistics in passing. This last category is more complex than the previous one, and so, as the aim of this book is to act as an introduction to key ideas in research, this section will be somewhat restricted, and simplified. More in-depth details can be gained from some of the many statistical texts available or statistics chapters in more advanced research books.

In simple terms, inferential statistics are used in two main ways. The first use is to estimate the probability that characteristics found in a sample accurately reflect those that may exist in the population as a whole. We will return to this in Chapter 14 on sampling; here, the point is that one of the basic assumptions of inferential statistics is that the sample has been drawn using probability sampling methods. This means the sample was chosen in such a way as to ensure it is reasonably representative of the larger group. If this has been achieved, then what we find in the sample should be found in a similar pattern in the larger population from which they have been drawn. The use of inferential statistics allows the researcher to indicate the probability that this match is true, within reasonable limits known as a confidence interval (CI). This is similar to the use of standard deviation, which is used in its construction, and gives and upper and lower limit between which the attribute or variable in which we are interested might lie in the larger population.

The second main use of inferential statistics is to help the researcher decide if the results of an experiment support the hypothesis that there is a difference between the experimental and control groups. This is achieved by being able to take an alternative hypothesis that there is no difference between the two groups, known as null-hypotheses (covered in the last chapter on experimental designs) and say that the difference found in the results between the two groups following the experiment is unlikely to support us saying that no difference exists. In other words, if there is a difference between the experimental and control groups it is more likely to be due to the intervention rather than simply to chance or some other explanation. This seems a very complicated procedure, but one that follows statistical logic and conventions. The hesitant language is due to the difficulty of designing the perfect and conclusive research study. As Burns and Grove (2009: 452) stress, 'Inferences are made cautiously and with great care', but statistical procedures allow us to provide some reassurance to support conclusions from well-designed experimental studies.

There are two types of inferential statistics: *parametric* and *non-parametric tests*. Parametric tests relate to the existence of real differences between experimental and control groups or the likelihood of characteristics in the sample being found in the wider population. However, they require a number of strict conditions to be met before they can be used. These include the following:

- The level of measurement applied to the variable must be interval or ratio (this is why understanding the levels of measurement is important).
- The distribution (spread) of the variable must be close to a normal distribution (spread evenly either side of the mean to form a bell shaped curve if plotted on a graph).
- The spread of the measurements should be uniformly close to the mean and not include a large number of 'outliers'. This condition is referred to as '*homogeneity of variance*'.

Despite these guidelines, the rules are sometimes broken on the assumption that these constraints are open to a certain amount of leeway. The advice for the novice, however, is that where there is any doubt about the features of the data, use non-parametric tests. For each parametric test there is a non-parametric equivalent so that the same calculation can be made; however, the strength of the relationship indicated by the test may be different.

A further distinction we can make regarding inferential statistics also divides into two main categories and they are: first, those that seek to establish a consistent pattern or *correlation* between two variables, and second, a group known as *tests of significance*, the latter of which are used to support or reject hypotheses.

CORRELATION

This statistical calculation explores the relationship between two variables collected from each person or item in a sample (e.g. width of pelvis and length of labour), and attempts to assess if they are related. It is important to stress it does not attempt to say that one causes the other, only that some kind of pattern or association exists between them. Correlation is an attempt to answer the question, to what extent are two variables related to each other in terms of *strength* – how closely are they related, and *direction* – whether they are positively related, that is, do measurements of both variables go up together or down together, or whether they are negatively related, that is, as one variable goes up the other goes down.

The strength of the relationship in correlation is measured by a *correlation coefficient*. This is a single number that is the product of a calculation that provides a measure of how closely the two variables are related. The correlation coefficient is measured on a scale between plus one (+1), which is a perfect *positive* correlation, and minus one (−1), a perfect *negative* correlation. When the calculation reveals that there is no relationship between two variables, the coefficient (the number that indicates the strength of the relationship) will be zero. In other words, we are dealing with a scale that looks something like Figure 13.2.

An illustration will clarify the way in which all correlations lie somewhere on the line in Figure 13.2. A perfect positive correlation between personal income and an individual's expenditure on clothes would mean that a 10% increase in income would result in an extra 10% increase in the amount spent on clothes. In the case of a negative correlation, it would mean that as measurements of one variable go up, for instance cost of travelling by train per kilometre, there would be a corresponding decrease in the number of rail passengers. A perfect negative correlation of −1 would be indicated when a 14% increase in the cost of rail fares per kilometre would result in a 14% drop in the number of passengers.

The important point about correlation is that it measures *similarities*, whereas tests of significance, which are used in RCTs, measure *differences*. This is a key principle in understanding the different purposes of these two statistical techniques. The usefulness of knowing a correlation exists is that it allows us to plan or make broad predictions that will be reasonably accurate, depending on the strength of the correlation. So, for instance, we know that there is a reasonably strong positive relationship between social class and the number of mothers who breastfeed. This means that if geographical areas are compared using a scale of social class, it can be expected that the demand for support for breastfeeding will be higher in those areas with a higher social class distribution. This kind of information, as Burns and Grove (2009) acknowledge, is crucial in planning modern health care delivery.

As there is rarely a perfect correlation between variables, a strong relationship will be anything from a value of 0.5 up to 0.8. A medium relationship will be around 0.3 to 0.4. A strong negative relationship, where the value of one variable goes up whilst another measure goes down, would be from −0.5 to −0.8. A useful checklist of correlation levels and their meaning is shown in Table 13.6.

Calculating correlation

There are two main methods of calculating correlation, depending on the type of data being examined. Where one of the variables is measured using an ordinal level of measurement, such as a Likert scale, or similar scale such as an Apgar score, where the precise difference between points on a scale is not known, then Spearman's rho (pronounced 'row') is used. This is indicated by

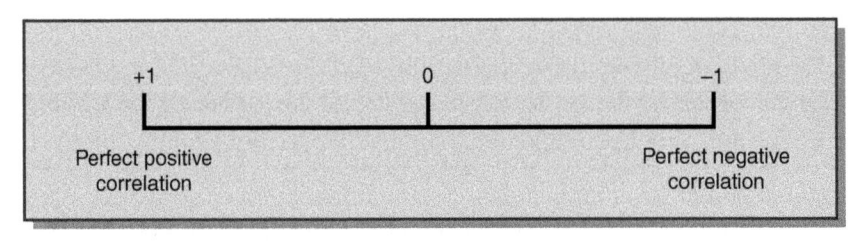

FIG 13.2 Scale used to indicate correlation coefficient.

Table 13.6 *Interpreting correlation*

Where the correlation coefficient is:	
0.9 to +1	A very strong to perfect positive correlation
0.5 up to 0.8	A good to strong positive relationship
0.3 or 0.4	A reasonable positive relationship
0 to 0.2	No to little evidence of a positive relationship
0 to −0.2	No to little evidence of a negative or inverse relationship
−0.3 or −0.4	A reasonable negative or inverse relationship
−0.5 to −0.8	A good to strong negative or inverse relationship
−0.9 to −1	A very strong to perfect negative or inverse correlation

the symbol r_s. If the measurements for both variables in a correlation are at interval or ratio level, and if they comply to a number of other stringent criteria, then a more accurate method called the Pearson product moment, usually referred to as Pearson r (or sometimes more informally as Pearson's r) is used.

Both measures use the same scale of between +1 and −1 to show the strength of the relationship between the two sets of measurements. Although Pearson r is a more accurate measurement, the nature of the measurements used in midwifery means that Spearman's rho may be more common.

Multiple regression

Before leaving correlation, it is worth mentioning a natural development of the technique, which is multiple regression. Whereas correlation works on the relationship between two variables, multiple regression takes the same idea but extends it to take into account at the same time a larger number of interval or ratio variables that might be related to a particular outcome.

TESTS OF SIGNIFICANCE

Tests of significance are crucial in clinical trials where researchers attempt to demonstrate that the intervention they introduced had an effect on a dependent variable (outcome). In choosing a test of significance researchers must ensure that the requirements for using the test are met by the data collected. Tests of significance can be either parametric or non-parametric. As indicated earlier, parametric tests provide the greatest degree of accuracy. A favourable statistical result using a parametric test indicates an important finding. However, the stringent conditions relating to the level of measurement and distribution of the data within the sample must be fulfilled before they can be accepted with confidence.

The conditions for using non-parametric tests are a lot easier to meet, and they can be used with much smaller data sets compared to parametric tests, but the degree of accuracy is less certain. In other words, the chances of being wrong in saying that real differences have been found between the groups in a study are greater when using a non-parametric test than when using a parametric equivalent. The difference between the data that can be used is again related to the level of measurement and also to whether the distribution of the variable meets the criteria of a normal distribution.

Some of the commonly encountered tests of significance are outlined in Table 13.7. Further details of these can be found in many of the statistics and research texts.

CONDUCTING RESEARCH

One of the inevitable demands on the quantitative researcher is to demonstrate an understanding of statistical techniques and the ability to use the right tests for the data collected. The method of analysis has to be considered at the design stage. As each item in the tool of data collection is chosen, the

Table 13.7 Common statistical tests and procedures you will encounter

Name of test	Type	Description
t-test Independent t-test Dependent t-test	Parametric test used on interval and ratio data.	The independent t-test is used to compare the means of two separate groups. The dependent t-test measures two means in the same group, using a 'before and after/pre-test post-test' design.
Mann–Whitney U test	Non-parametric equivalent of the t-test.	Used to compare the means of two groups with ordinal data, where data are not normally distributed.
Wilcoxon test	The non-parametric equivalent of the dependent t-test.	Used where scores are in pairs, such as pre-test post-test design, but where data are not normally distributed.
Chi-squared test (χ^2)	Non-parametric test The simple χ^2 uses nominal data, the complex χ^2 is used where there are three or more sets of data.	Looks at whether the difference between two groups was as expected. Are the groups the same or different? Applies to nominal or ordinal data.
Pearson coefficient (Pearson r)	Parametric test that establishes the relationship between two interval or ratio variables.	The size of the relationship is indicated on a scale between +1 and −1. Strong relationships are usually around 0.5 to 0.8 positive or negative.
Spearman's coefficient Spearman's rho ('row') r	This is the non-parametric version of the above and is used with nominal or ordinal data.	As above.

researcher should consider the level of measurement that will be required. The basic principle is to collect data at the highest level practical, for example, specific age should be collected rather than grouped data (ordinal) or even nominal level, e.g. below 21, or 21 to 25, unless it is known for sure that calculations such as mean, median or standard deviation will not be required. Collecting data at the highest level ensures a greater choice in data presentation and analysis and greater accuracy of the results.

Consulting other researchers' findings is helpful in deciding how you might present information, such as in the form of a table or other visual display. You must also consider whether some variables need to be cross-tabulated with other items of information. I have often constructed 'dummy' tables at this point to explore the different ways data might be displayed. Decide which variables will be shown as columns and which in rows as well as the direction in which percentages will be calculated (row percentages or column percentages). The appropriate statistical calculations or tests can also be written alongside the dummy tables to remind you at a later stage.

The level of measurement will influence the options available for presentation, especially where graphical presentations are concerned. So, for instance, nominal- and ordinal-level data can be shown as a table, but are often clearer as a bar chart or pie chart. Interval- and ratio-level data can be displayed as a histogram, but not as a bar chart, as they are suitable for continuous data. Line graphs can also be used for interval and ratio data.

At the data input stage, the data from the raw questionnaires, observation checklists, etc. will be entered on the computer. Quality control of data inputting should be built in to the process, especially where more than one person is involved in entering the data. The random checking of data entered is worthwhile to confirm accuracy and pick up errors. Unfortunately, there is nothing similar to a spell checker to pick up errors in typing numbers; they all have to be checked against the originals.

One of the first tasks of the data analysis stage is to summarise the data ready for statistical processing. Summarising can be as simple as counting how many times options were chosen or occurred in a frequency distribution. This is carried out on the characteristics of the sample, such as age, parity, grade of staff, or whatever sample characteristics have been collected. At the planning stage, the grouping or banding of some data might need to take place, so, for instance, lengths of time or age may be grouped (remembering the points made earlier on levels of measurement). The size of the bandings can be determined from previous research, but it is worth noting that too small a banding can lead to information overload and hide broader patterns; too large a banding will lose the sensitivity of some data in highlighting differences amongst smaller groupings.

One major error to avoid in grouping categories is overlapping the groups. Taking the example of age, there is no point in having one group 20 to 25 and then the next group 25 to 30, as 25 appears twice. It should be 20 to 25 then 26 to 30 and so on.

Once the data have been processed they can be selectively turned into visual displays. Most computers are now capable of producing tables and, through spreadsheet programmes such as Excel©, can present their content in a number of appropriate forms such as bar charts and pie charts. As with other aspects of the research process, it is important to pay attention to detail. Look at this aspect of the research as a crucial part of getting your points across. Unless the statistical elements in your research have been carried out professionally, and to a high standard, the credibility of your results will suffer.

CRITIQUING RESEARCH

The purpose of this chapter has been to help you become more familiar with a small number of the basic ideas behind statistical analysis and forms of data presentation. These are most commonly encountered in the results sections of research papers or presentations. The immediate reaction of many people confronted by statistics is to panic. This is an emotional response that can be controlled. The information in this chapter has hopefully helped you to realise there is a logic and order to statistics that can be appreciated and understood, and you do not have to know it all.

When faced with a quantitative researcher paper, the first thing to do is to look very carefully at the labels attached to the tables and figures. What do they show? Then look at how this information is presented to you, and begin to read the story it reveals. Look at tables or figures and ask yourself, 'Are these descriptive or inferential statistics?' If they are descriptive, you will need to examine the size of categories. How big was the study, is there a pattern to the frequencies across the categories (which categories have the biggest numbers attached to them, which have the smallest)? Would you have anticipated the size of these? Look at the relative size between the categories. Is there a slow step down in size or are there one or two large categories, and then a big drop in size before the next categories?

Whether it is a table or diagram, can you read the story of what is going on? What does it suggest to you? Are there questions raised in your mind as a result of the pattern you see? Where inferential statistics are used, look in or below the table, where there should be additional information such as the tests that have been carried out and the 'p' values that have been produced. This may even be in the methods sections under 'statistical analysis', or where the results are described. What does the size of these values suggest to you? The closer the 'p' value is to 1, the more likely the null-hypothesis is to be correct and there is no difference between groups or variables; the closer it is to zero (starting from a value of $p<0.05$ and getting smaller) the more likely the alternative hypothesis of a real difference between the groups produced by the independent variable is to be true.

In the case of an RCT, has the author demonstrated statistically that the groups were comparable to start? If not, is there anything about the differences that could play a part in interpreting the results? Similarly, in the case of an RCT, could the numbers dropping out of any of the groups have made a difference to the meaningful comparisons between the groups?

Once you have searched the figures and tables for meaning, read through the text to see what the writer makes of all this. Do they talk you through the tables and point out things that you may not have noticed, or explained what the results suggested to them? Where the data raised questions in your mind, do the authors answer those questions for you? Where there are unfamiliar statistical elements or things you have forgotten, check them out in this chapter or in a more advanced statistics reference book. Depending on where the article is published, you may feel questions such as whether the authors have used appropriate statistical procedures or tests should have been established by the journal. Be aware that this is not true of all journals.

Do not ignore tables and figures. Do try and get something out of them. Each time you do this thorough analysis, you will learn a little bit more, and become more relaxed about reading the statistical elements in a study.

KEY POINTS

- Collecting quantitative data means that statistical processes will be involved in the analysis stage. Understanding the principles behind these processes is important in correctly interpreting the findings of research.
- Research findings are presented following certain conventions and use presentation methods such as tables, bar charts, histograms and pie charts. Every picture tells a story, so these should never be overlooked.
- Statistics fall into two main categories of descriptive and inferential. Users of research need to know the principles and assumptions on which these are based as well as those relating to parametric and non-parametric tests.
- The level of measurement of the data will influence many of the decisions made in the research process. An understanding of these levels is crucial to understanding why certain decisions are made in the choice of statistical techniques.
- Although the jargon and symbols used in statistics may look intimidating, in reality a basic understanding is not difficult to achieve. Competency in understanding basic statistical principles is essential to applying research to evidence-based practice.

REFERENCES

Atkinson, I., 2008. Descriptive statistics. In: Watson, R., McKenna, H., Cowman, S., Keady, J. (Eds.), Nursing Research: Designs and Methods. Churchill Livingstone, Edinburgh.

Burns, N., Grove, S., 2009. The Practice of Nursing Research: Appraisal, Synthesis, and Generation of Evidence. sixth ed. Saunders, St Louis.

McDonald, S., Henderson, J., Faulkner, S., Evans, S., Hagan, R., 2010. Effect of an extended midwifery postnatal support programme on the duration of breast feeding: A randomised controlled trial. Midwifery 26 (1), 88–100.

Polit, D., Beck, C., 2008. Nursing Research: Generating and Assessing Evidence for Nursing Practice. eighth ed. Lippincott Williams and Wilkins, Philadelphia.

Spiby, H., Munro, J. (Eds.), 2010. Evidence Based Midwifery: Applications in Context. Wiley-Blackwell, Chichester.

Walters, S., Freeman, J., 2010. Descriptive analysis of quantitative data. In: Gerrish, K., Lacey, A. (Eds.), The Research Process in Nursing, sixth ed. Wiley-Blackwell, Chichester.

Sampling methods

14

The outcome of any research project is dependent on both the reliability and validity of the data collection method used, and the type and quality of the sample on which the results are based. Sampling is an area of research that contains a number of specialised words and ideas that require attention. In this chapter the issues relating to who or what is included in the sample, and the alternative methods for choosing the sample, known as sampling strategies, will be examined.

It is useful to clarify the difference between a *'population'* and *'sample'* as these are two common terms used in sampling. Although these terms appear to be used almost interchangeably, there is a clear difference between them. The population is the total group of people, things or events the researcher is interested in saying something about, e.g. midwives who have a higher degree, women who have a home birth. Schmidt and Brown (2009) refer to this as the 'target population'. The sample is a section of those from the population who are accessed to provide data to answer the study aim. The main issue is to select the sample so that they resemble the main population closely enough to provide similar answers or measurements to those that might have been produced by the whole group. The method of selecting the sample is a key methodological issue in research. This selection method is called the *sampling strategy* and describes the process of choosing individuals, events, behaviours or elements for participation in a study (Burns and Grove 2009). There are a number of ways of arriving at a sample. The choice will vary depending on whether the research approach is:

- experimental,
- survey,
- qualitative.

The choice of sampling strategy will be influenced by how far the researcher wants to generalise, that is, apply the findings to the wider population. The more important it is to achieve a close fit between the sample and the population, the more complex the sampling strategy used. Whatever the purpose of the study, the researcher is faced with three vital questions:

- *Who* or what will make up the sample?
- *How* will they be chosen?
- *How many* will be chosen?

The remainder of the chapter will illustrate the way in which these questions are answered.

WHY SAMPLE?

Why bother to sample in the first place? Surely it must be more accurate to get information from a total group? True, but in terms of practicalities, it will not always be possible to collect information from an entire group. For example, we cannot send a questionnaire to every pregnant woman in Britain as many would have given birth before we found out who should be included. It can also be extremely expensive to gather information from a total group, and it may not always be that much more accurate than a sample. The solution is to select a sample from the population in such a way that the process creates the minimum of bias and represents the characteristics of those in the population as closely as possible. A biased sample would consist of people, events or things that were very different from those in the total group. An example of a biased sample would be a group of pregnant midwives who are asked how they intended feeding their baby. We would expect there to be a difference between this sample and the total population of pregnant women; this would make decisions based on the results unreliable.

It is clear from this that the method of sampling deserves a great deal of thought. We should ensure that it has been planned in such a way as to recognise and minimise potential bias.

INCLUSION/EXCLUSION CRITERIA

Before we select our sample we need to define our target population accurately. This is achieved by specifying *inclusion* and *exclusion criteria*. Inclusion criteria are the characteristics we want those in our sample to possess. This is why it is sometimes referred to as *eligibility criteria* (Polit and Beck 2008). Examples of inclusion criteria would be women who have a normal vaginal birth at term, or women in certain age groups with no complications of pregnancy. In other words, it is the characteristics they *must* possess to allow them to stand for the general group we want to say something about.

Exclusion criteria consist of those characteristics we do not want those in our sample to possess because it may make them untypical and so bias the results. There may be other reasons for excluding some people from a study, such as the risk of harm for those with a certain medical condition or characteristics.

The researcher must consider the inclusion and exclusion criteria at the planning stage, as these will form part of the detail put into a *research proposal* or outline of an intended piece of research. These details will also be included in any final report and allow the reader to consider whether the criteria could lead to some limitations in applying the results to other groups. Clear examples of inclusion and exclusion criteria are usually found in randomised control trials (RCTs) that are very sensitive to bias. So, for example, the following appears in the study by McDonald et al. (2010: 90), who looked at the provision of extra support for women following birth to establish influences on length of time breastfeeding:

> *Women who had given birth at King Edward Memorial Hospital (KEMH), Perth, Western Australia, and who intended to breast feed were eligible for entry into the trial. ... Exclusion criteria were: gestational age less than 36 completed weeks; multiple pregnancy; maternal age less than 18 years; and insufficient English to complete questionnaires. Women who lived outside the Perth metropolitan area or who were not contactable by telephone were also excluded.*

SAMPLING METHODS

Different research approaches will require different sampling methods, although some methods can be used in a variety of approaches. In any situation, the researcher must try to draw the sample in such a way as to:

- reduce sampling bias,
- increase representativeness.

Sampling bias, according to Polit and Beck (2008: 340), is 'the systematic over-representation or under-representation of some segment of the population in terms of a characteristic relevant to the research question'. Where bias is avoided, or minimised, there is a greater chance that the results can be applied to situations other than the one in which the data were gathered. In other words, it is easier to generalise from the results.

Bias is reduced if the researcher can increase the representativeness of those chosen for the sample. They should match the population they represent as closely as possible in the ways that might influence the outcome of the study. This would include variables such as parity, social class, age and education level. The researcher should establish the distribution of such variables in the population and then demonstrate statistically that the sample does not differ significantly from the total group in the possession of those characteristics.

Table 14.1 outlines the main sampling strategies linked to the various broad research approaches, as there are some clear differences in sampling methods and sample sizes between quantitative and qualitative approaches.

EXPERIMENTAL SAMPLING APPROACHES

As we saw in Chapter 12, experiments play a key role in establishing the presence of cause-and-effect relationships between variables. To achieve this, sampling must be carried out in very meticulous way so that an accurate conclusion can be deduced from the results. The method of sampling is drawn from a number of options grouped under the heading of *random sampling methods*. These options form what are called *probability sampling* methods. Using this approach, every unit in the population, whether it is people, things or events, should have an equal chance of being selected. If this criterion is

Table 14.1 *Sampling method by broad research approach*

Research approach	Sampling method
Experimental	Simple random Stratified sampling Proportionate random
Quasi-experimental and ex post facto	Comparative groups Systematic random
Survey	Simple random Stratified random Proportionate random Systematic random Opportunity/convenience/accidental Quota
Qualitative	Purposive Opportunity/convenience/accidental Snowball/network/chain/nominated Theoretical

achieved, it means that some of the more sophisticated statistical tests can be applied to the results. These allow the accuracy of statements made about the results to be calculated. Some of the alternative sampling methods in experimental design are:

- simple random sample,
- stratified sample,
- proportionate sampling.

SIMPLE RANDOM SAMPLE

In many experimental situations it is not possible or desirable to enlist a whole population in the study, and a simple random sampling design is used instead. This is perhaps one of the most commonly misunderstood concepts in sampling. Many people assume that choosing a random sample is a haphazard, casual or indiscriminate way of selecting people for a study. The word 'random' is assumed to imply that there is very little system applied to this process, which is far from the truth.

One essential distinction is between a *random sample* and *random allocation*. In a random sample those eligible to be included in the study are identified from the larger population, and are selected for inclusion in the research. This does not mean they have agreed to be included in the study, or that they will willingly take part. In the view of some researchers, findings can only be generalised if random sampling has taken place.

Random allocation is frequently used in health service experimental research; it is the system by which individuals who have agreed to take part in a study are allocated to either the experimental or control group so that there is minimum bias surrounding who ends up in which group. There is no guarantee that those who agree to take part in a random allocation research project are similar to the wider population. In fact, those who agree to take part in research may be very different from the general population.

In order to achieve a random sample, the researcher must have a complete list, or *sampling frame*, of all those who could be accessed to take part in the study, that is, the *study population*. A sampling frame can be defined as a list of the study population who meet the inclusion and exclusion criteria of the study. Procter et al. (2010) stress that the sampling frame consists of those in the study population, that is, those the researcher can access, not the target population, that is, those who form the bigger group that study wants to say something about. The study population should naturally mirror the target population as closely as possible. So women who have had a previous Caesarean section may be the target population, and those who have had a previous Caesarean section in one local maternity unit in the last 5 years will be the study population. Once the frame is constructed, individuals are consecutively given a number to identify them for the purposes of sample selection.

Individuals are then selected for inclusion in the study using a table of random numbers or list of computer-generated random numbers. Box 14.1 illustrates a small portion of a table of random numbers. These can be found in many research textbooks, books on statistics, or book of random number tables. In all such tables, there is no systematic sequence or order to the way in which the numbers are listed. That is, they do not go up or down in any particular pattern, or are listed in an alternating odd/even way.

Using a table of random numbers

How do we randomly allocate people in an experiment? Let us imagine the researcher has gained the agreement of 50 women and has decided to allocate 25 to an experimental group and 25 to the control group. A sampling frame of the names of the 50 women is first constructed. The order of the names is not important. Everyone is given a number in sequence from 1 to 50. Then 25 numbers between 1 and 50 are extracted from the table of random numbers to form the experimental group. The remaining 25 women whose numbers have not been picked will form the control group.

BOX 14.1 Example of a part of a table of random numbers										
12	57	42	14	01	84	35	21	75	33	61	68	32
85	83	35	22	13	38	47	90	15	65	74	40	09
10	39	55	86	16	03	91	75	62	34	11	59	17
22	08	60	13	26	99	71	40	91	69	35	04	65
49	74	26	39	09	16	87	56	20	54	88	93	82
36	06	33	47	98	49	07	19	51	27	43	71	54

The method of selecting the numbers can now be described. Without looking closely at the table of random numbers, the researcher puts a finger down on to the page and looks for the number closest to it. For the purpose of illustration, let us say the number 83 has been identified. This is the second number in the second column in Box 14.1. As this is above 50, which is the number of people who have been allocated a number, it is ignored. Keeping the finger on the page, the researcher now moves their finger, right, left, up or down, or diagonally in any direction. As the finger is moved, each number between 1 and 50 is accepted and any above 50 rejected. If a number has already been selected it is also rejected until 25 different numbers have been drawn. So let us assume, having started at 83, we continue to move in a straight line to the right along the row. This would give us numbers 35, 22, 13, 38 and 47. Number 90 would be rejected, and 15 accepted. At any point the researcher may alter direction, or lift the finger and replace it at a different point. It really does not matter.

Once the 25 numbers have been drawn, those people who have been allocated each of those numbers will be identified from the sampling frame. These will form the people in the experimental group. Anyone with a number not included in the 25 drawn at random would be in the control group.

How would this work in the case of an RCT where a sampling frame could not be constructed? For example, if people were to be selected for a prospective study as they entered the system, say at a booking clinic? In this case the researcher would use sealed envelopes. The table of random numbers would be used in the same way as just described where, if the researcher again wished to use two groups of 25 women, 25 numbers would be picked out and designated the experimental group. A pack of envelopes would then be numbered from 1 to 50. In those envelopes whose number corresponded with one of the 25 numbers drawn from the random table, a slip of paper saying 'Group A' (which, unbeknown to the person, would indicate the experimental group) or stating what had been designated as the experimental intervention would be placed in the envelope. All the other envelopes would have a slip indicating 'Group B' (the control group) or the control intervention, or no intervention where an experimental variable was being compared to no intervention.

The envelopes would then be placed in number sequence from 1 to 50. As each person who had agreed to take part entered the study, the researcher would open the next envelope in sequence, and follow the instructions. The use of 'A' or 'B' would 'blind' them to which group the individual had been allocated.

In the example of a table of random numbers, it should be clear that the table used would only be applicable if the total number of people in the sampling frame held a maximum of a 99. For larger studies, it is possible to join pairs of figures in a table together or to computer generate numbers with three digit numbers that would be applicable for sampling frames extending up to 999.

STRATIFIED SAMPLE

The basic principle of a simple random sample is that everyone has an equal chance of being allocated to either the experimental or control group. There are cases, however, where this method may result in an over-representation of certain characteristics in one of the groups. So, for instance, the experimental group could have mainly primigravida women and the control group mainly multigravida women and this may have a distorting effect on the outcome measure, as labour in each group can be different.

To avoid this, the researcher can first stratify the sample into parity and then sample each parity group appropriately. In the case of a prospective experimental design, the researcher would use numbered envelopes for each parity group. Once it is established whether the individual agreeing to take part in the study is primigravida or multigravida, the next envelope in the appropriate pile is opened. This way there should be an even spread of each parity group in both the experimental and control group.

PROPORTIONATE SAMPLING

A further refinement of the stratified sample is the proportionate sample. Here, the number of participants should be selected in proportion to their occurrence in the population (Burns and Grove 2009). So, with the example of parity, it could be felt important that the sample should reflect the proportion of primigravida to multigravida women within each experimental and control group. If there were a proportion of 60% multigravida women birthing in a particular clinical area to 40% primigravida, then a proportional sample would also provide a sample with the same ratio between parities.

QUASI-EXPERIMENTAL AND EX POST FACTO DESIGNS

Chapter 12 discussed a number of alternatives to RCTs, such as quasi-experimental and ex post facto designs. Quasi-experimental designs are used where it is not possible, usually for reasons such as ethical difficulties or practical constraints, to randomly allocate people to experimental and control groups. In these circumstances, groups already formed are used. Examples would be women on two different wards, or couples attending two different locations for antenatal education. One location is used for the experimental group, and the other for the control group and the results from both groups compared.

The difficulty of this design is that it is not possible to rule out bias due to the blend of characteristics or experiences in each group. In other words, there may be important differences within the groups that may influence the outcome following an experimental intervention. Although this is a fundamental sampling weakness, in many cases this choice of design is the only one available. In these circumstances, the researcher will attempt to illustrate the comparability between the two groups by identifying and describing key demographic characteristics, such as age, parity, social class.

As there is an unequal difference in the chance of people ending up in the experimental as opposed to the control group (everyone on one ward would have a 100% chance and those on the comparison or control ward would have 0% chance), this is known as a non-probability sampling method. This is not as accurate a means of detecting true differences between groups as a probability sampling method, and for this reason non-probability sampling methods are less respected than probability methods. However, a non-probability sampling method has the advantage of being practical and often the best that can be done under the circumstances.

Ex post facto studies, also discussed in Chapter 12, are very similar to the quasi-experimental approach in the sampling methods used. The term means 'after the fact' and relates to the formation of groups that have already taken place before the start of the study and differ in relation to the independent variable. The researcher does not introduce the variable, but searches for groups or individuals who share a common identity on the basis of their own past decision to adopt a characteristic, such as smoking, or behaviour, such as deciding to breastfeed. Again, this is a non-probability method and we cannot generalise the findings to other situations with the same confidence as we can with probability sampling methods.

SURVEY METHODS

Although experimental designs are important to support evidence-based practice, a far more frequently used approach to research in midwifery is that of the survey. Here, some of the sampling methods already mentioned can be used and fall into both the probability and non-probability sampling methods.

SIMPLE RANDOM SAMPLING

Surveys are very powerful where they are based on a simple random sample. Here, everyone from the study population has an equal chance of being included in the survey. The method has been described above under experiments, where a sampling frame containing everyone fitting the inclusion criteria is constructed; a table of random numbers is then used to pick out the appropriate number of individuals for inclusion in the survey.

The advantage of using this method is that it is possible to make generalisations concerning the wider population on the basis of a random sample. This is because it falls into the category of probability sampling methods. One disadvantage of this method, however, is the difficulty of constructing a suitable sampling frame where there are a large number of eligible individuals in the target population, or where no list of likely individuals exists.

STRATIFIED SAMPLING

The process of simple random sampling in surveys can be refined further by dividing those eligible to be included in the sample into appropriate strata and then sampling from within each of the groups created. Examples of this would include grouping women by parity, or in the case of midwives, grade, or length of experience.

The advantage of a stratified sample is that it ensures that those from relevant subgroups are included in the study. The disadvantages include the difficulty of predicting which subgroups might make a difference to the outcome, and then the problem of dividing the sampling frame into those characteristics. For instance, if it was thought that women with high self-esteem were more likely to breastfeed in relation to those with medium or low self-esteem, it would be difficult first to divide the target group into strata by level of self-confidence without the prior use of a scale measuring self-esteem.

PROPORTIONATE SAMPLING

Proportionate sampling in a survey would be an attempt to construct subgroups within the sample that were similar in proportion to the broader population. The aim would be to ensure that an unrepresentative proportion in one group did not produce a biased result. An example would be a survey of midwives' views on a particular aspect of midwifery. To ensure that the influence of grade was kept constant, the population would first be stratified according to grade; then the numbers selected from each group would mirror the proportion in each grade in the total population. Again, this example would use a sampling frame and table of random numbers, or computer generated random numbers. The advantage of this approach is a greater chance of accuracy and reduction in bias. The problems are similar to stratified sampling, and that is the difficulty of having prior knowledge of the size and location of some of the subgroups.

SYSTEMATIC SAMPLING

In some surveys where individuals or objects are being selected for inclusion from a very large study population, systematic sampling is used in order to gain elements across the entire population. This is achieved by numbering all those who fit the inclusion criteria, then using a table of random numbers. The first number is selected randomly, and then the subsequent individuals would be selected following a predetermined frequency, such as every fifth, tenth or, with very long lists every, twentieth, fiftieth or even one-hundredth person or object.

The *sampling interval*, that is, the distance between each unit in the sample, can be determined by first deciding on the total number required in the sample and then dividing that into the total number in the group. An example would be a questionnaire given to a sample of women who had delivered in a particular unit over a 3-year period. If it was decided that the sample size required should be 80, and there were 3472 deliveries, then dividing that number by 80 would give a sampling interval of every forty-third person.

In order to ensure that women from the whole of the 3 years were represented, all those discharged could be numbered, using a table of random numbers, the first number could be drawn out, for example 33, and then every forty-third number following that in the sampling frame would be chosen. This would include number 33, then 76, 119, 162 and so on, to provide an even spread across the 3 years. Because the first number had been chosen randomly, it would still conform to the criteria of a probability sample.

CLUSTER SAMPLING

Where the elements in the sampling frame are geographically spread, or where the individual elements making up a population are unknown, a multistage approach called cluster sampling can be used (Burns and Grove 2009).

Imagine a national survey of the opinions of GPs regarding how they perceived the role of the midwife in providing care for women in the community. A sampling frame of all GPs would be a tall order; instead, the researchers may first produce a sampling frame of all health regions within Britain, and randomly select, say, a sample of 10 regions. For each region, they could then construct a sampling frame of districts. From this a total of three districts from each area might be chosen. The final sampling frame might be a list of all GP practices within the districts randomly chosen. From this a final total of 20 GP practices could be randomly chosen and every GPs in those practices sent questionnaires.

It is clear from this example why it is called *multistage sampling*. At each stage a sampling frame is constructed, and a simple random sample selected. Each level consists of the construction of the next sampling frame until the size of the units is manageable, at which point everyone in the group is included. The advantage of this system is that it can achieve an accessible sample from an almost impossible total population. This reduces costs, as those included are found close together, making access and communication easier and also making a probability method possible where a sampling frame with each person listed is difficult to achieve (Proctor et al. 2010). The disadvantage is that the number of layers to the sampling process increases the danger of not arriving at a truly representative sample, and is considered not to be as accurate as simple random or stratified sampling (Polit and Beck 2008).

CONVENIENCE/OPPORTUNITY/ACCIDENTAL SAMPLING

These three terms are often used to describe the same approach to sampling where the researcher includes in the study those people to whom they have easy access, and who happen to be in the right place at the right time. Here, the researcher selects the most easily accessible people from the population. This is the method used by market researchers where people are stopped in the street and asked to answer questions. It is this method that people frequently mistake for a random sample.

Along with the next two methods described below, this approach falls into the category of a non-probability sampling method, as everyone does not have the same chance of being included. There is no way of knowing whether those in this type of sample are representative of the larger group. The ability to generalise from the findings is consequently restricted. Nevertheless, these approaches continue to be very popular because they are very pragmatic in gaining quick and easy access to a sample, and provide an indication of possible responses to questions.

Examples of convenience samples might be women attending a particular antenatal clinic on a certain day, or midwives attending a study day who might be asked their opinions on some midwifery issue. The relevance of terms such as convenience or opportunity can be clearly seen from these examples.

One further example of a convenience sample is the self-selecting sample, who are people who volunteer to take part in a study, for example, by returning a questionnaire or responding to a poster or advertisement to take part in a survey. Examples can be found in both magazines and professional journals. This is far from an ideal method as there is little the researcher can do to ensure that those returning questionnaires are typical and so there is always the possibility of bias of an unknown size.

In summary, the advantage of the convenience sampling approach is that it is simple, cheap, and quick and does not require the construction of elaborate sampling frames. The main disadvantage is sampling bias, in that those who happen to be around a particular location or in one particular group may not be typical of the wider population they represent. The same is true for those who self-select themselves into a survey, especially those for magazines and journals. Polit and Beck (2008) agree and warn that non-probability samples are rarely representative of the target population, as some segments of the population are likely to be systematically under-represented. An important point, however, is the extent to which there is variation in the population of the variable being studied, where the variation in a certain variable in the population is small, forming a homogenous group, the risk of bias may be low, but where it is a very mixed or heterogeneous population the risk of bias is greater.

QUOTA SAMPLING

This method is a refinement of convenience sampling and attempts to produce a sample that is similar in certain key characteristics to the total population. The market researcher will use quota sampling by selecting so many people in certain age groups or occupation groups in order to argue that the sample is 'similar in structure' to the total population. In midwifery, there may be a similar attempt to include quotas such as so many women who are primigravida and so many multigravida, or in various age groups, or have experienced certain types of labour.

In many respects, quota sampling is similar in purpose to stratified sampling, but it differs from a stratified sample in that the participants are not randomly selected from each strata. The advantage of quota sampling is that the researcher is in a stronger position to say that because the sample is similar to the total population, then the results may be reasonably representative. The disadvantages are similar to stratified sampling, in that there is an assumption that the subgroupings that may make a difference to the results are already known, and that the size of each of the groups is also known so that the size of the quotas can be calculated. It also depends on the information that allocates respondents to either one quota or another being easily ascertained from potential respondents.

Surveys, then, can be based on a variety of sampling methods. Some of these will result in statistical precision where probability sampling methods have been used. Where these are employed, reasonably large samples may be sought and chosen from the wider population using random sampling approaches based on accurate sampling frames. The aim of this kind of survey is to be able to generalise the results to the wider population. Other approaches based on non-probability sampling methods are less precise, but a lot easier to conduct. Although it is difficult to judge their accuracy, they can provide useful 'snapshots' of situations that can be used as the basis for action.

QUALITATIVE APPROACHES

As qualitative research differs in so many respects from quantitative research, it is no surprise that the approach to sampling is also different. Because the aim is not to achieve a large representative sample from which generalisations can be made, sampling is not based on probability methods. The aim is rather to gather information from people who can provide inside information on specific kinds of experiences or who are part of a particular culture or subgroup. In terms of inclusion criteria, the most important factor is that they have knowledge or experience of the topic or phenomenon under examination. Those who are part of a qualitative study do not 'stand for' the larger population, in the same way as in quantitative research; they are included on the basis that they are members of an appropriate group. However, there is an attempt in many studies to get a cross-section of representative people. On the whole, as Holloway and Wheeler (2010) note, the rules of qualitative sampling are less rigid that those of quantitative methods, where a strict sampling frame is established before the research starts. The main choices of sampling methods in qualitative research include:

- purposive,
- convenience,
- snowball/network/chain/nominated sample,
- theoretical.

PURPOSIVE SAMPLING

This alternative, also known as *judgemental sampling*, involves the researcher handpicking those in the sample on the basis of the researcher's knowledge of characteristics they know the individual possesses. It can also refer to the location or setting of the study (Holloway and Wheeler 2010). Although this seems likely to result in a biased sample, its aim is to achieve the opposite, by ensuring that a range of opinions or experiences is included.

The advantages of this method are that the sample is known to possess key characteristics that should be included in the survey; it is very practical and efficient in terms of time and money. The disadvantage is clearly that we are dependent on the researcher's judgement, which cannot be checked.

CONVENIENCE SAMPLE

Just as the purposive sample provides the researcher with relevant information, so the convenience sample within qualitative research is relevant as long as those at hand have the necessary information or experience relevant to the purpose of the study. The convenience sample can be used in both phenomenological studies and ethnographic research where the researcher draws on the experiences and activities of those who just happen to be in the setting being observed or under study. The appropriateness of this method again illustrates the flexibility in this approach to data collection.

SNOWBALL/NETWORK/CHAIN/NOMINATED SAMPLING

All of these terms describe the situation where the researcher identifies individuals with the necessary characteristics or experiences, and then asks them to suggest others who may be willing to participate in the study. Holloway and Wheeler (2010) point out that this kind of sampling method is used where the researcher finds it difficult to identify useful informants. This can take a number of forms such as individuals who cannot be easily contacted, or where individuals hide characteristics for fear that an undesirable label may be attached to them, e.g. mothers who are illicit drug takers. In many of these cases sampling frames just do not exist.

Burns and Grove (2009) point out that the advantage of this method is that 'nominated' friends tend to have characteristics in common and therefore it is a good way to collect a sample of people who share the characteristic under study. They go on to warn that biases are built into this sampling procedure, as subjects are not independent of each other. This may not, however, be a problem. However, such a method may miss those who are isolated from a social network and therefore such views may be missing from our developing knowledge-base.

THEORETICAL SAMPLING

Theoretical sampling is frequently used in grounded theory (Chapter 4) as a way of selecting the sample, and as a way of guiding the decision to stop data gathering. This is based on the principle that those in the sample can provide examples and insights into the concepts or theoretical issues that underpin the study. This helps to determine who will be included in the sample and if further individuals may help shed light on the issues pursued and contribute to completing the theory being developed (Burns and Grove 2009). Data collection continues until no new insights are gained, and there is a repetition of information already gained. This is called *theoretical saturation*. At this point, data collection stops.

SAMPLE SIZE

One of the most difficult tasks for the researcher at the planning stage is to estimate how many people, things or events are going to be included in the sample. As the type of study, to a large extent, influences the size of a sample, it is useful to consider the question of size under each of the headings already used in this chapter.

EXPERIMENTAL DESIGNS

As experimental designs are concerned with accuracy, there are some statistical guidelines the researcher can use in choosing a suitable sample size. The important factor is the size of the difference the researcher is looking for between the results of the experimental group and the control group before it can be said that an intervention has been successful. Unfortunately, for many conditions or situations, the difference between one group and another when measured on physiological outcomes may be quite small. This would mean that for differences to show up, the study would have to include quite a large number of people before that difference was clearly visible and statistically relevant. This is why, in medical research, the size of the sample can run into hundreds and sometimes even thousands.

The statistical procedure of *power analysis* can be used to estimate the total size of the sample needed, given an anticipated difference in the results between two groups (Proctor et al. 2010). However, in midwifery the number of experimental studies is relatively small, and some of those undertaken can be quite modest in sample size. It is often practical considerations such as time and resources that dictate the size of experimental groups. Closely examining the literature for the size of previous studies can be a great help to the researcher in estimating possible sample size. It is also important to realise that it is not so much the total number of people to be admitted to a trial that is important, but the size of the subgroups used in the analysis of the results. Where the sample is divided into different subgroups such as parity or age, the size of the groups can be quite small, even though at the start the overall sample might have been quite large.

One problem in experimental designs is the dropout rate from the study. This is referred to as *sample mortality* or *attrition*. Although the size of the sample can seem large to start, if the study is carried out over a long time period, or consists of several periods of testing and data collection, there can be a number of people who leave the study. This can have consequences where there is a larger proportion dropping out of one of the groups, as it can lead to an imbalance in the characteristics of the experimental and control group members so that they may no longer be comparable. The best the researcher can do is to try to make the size of the groups as large as is practical, and to ensure that the size is reasonably in line with any previous research.

SURVEYS

The optimum sample size in surveys is variable, as it relates to the size of the total population. In surveys where the aim is to be able to generalise quite accurately to the total population, the sample size might be in the hundreds, but in other studies, where the total population itself is quite small, such as the number of male midwives, the sample might be quite small.

In choosing the sample size, the advice is to gain as large a sample as possible on the grounds that the larger the sample, the more representative it is likely to be (Polit and Beck 2008: 348). However, there is also agreement that a large sample does not compensate for poor sampling methods. The ultimate criterion for assessing is the extent to which those include are clearly representative of the target sample group. In other words, the researcher should be concerned with the quality of the sampling method and the extent to which it avoids bias, rather than simply including as large a number as possible.

As with experimental studies, it is often practical considerations that influence sample size. These include time, money and the availability of subjects. The researcher should also consider the extent to which the variables included in the survey vary in the population. The more something varies, the larger the sample needed to gather a range of responses. The less something varies, the easier it is to capture the range of experience or opinion with a smaller sample.

QUALITATIVE RESEARCH

As we have seen throughout this and other chapters, qualitative research is so different from quantitative research that different considerations exist in almost all elements of the study, including sample size. Holloway and Wheeler (2010) note that sample size in qualitative research is not an indicator of the importance of the study or the quality of the findings, and point out that generally qualitative samples consist of fairly small numbers with anything from

4 to 50 participants. Although larger numbers are possible, they are not common. It is more usual to find much smaller numbers such as the 10 midwives included in the study by Byrom and Downe (2010) that explored midwives' accounts of the characteristics of 'good' leadership and 'good' midwifery. A somewhat larger study by Huber and Sandall (2009) explored the relationship between a one-to-one model of maternity care and the creation of calm during labour. The sample here included ten women, seven of their birth partners, and four midwives. Although both of these studies would appear too small within a quantitative paradigm, within the qualitative paradigm the sample size is wholly appropriate to provide a rich and enlightening study.

CONDUCTING RESEARCH

In conducting a research project there are some important decisions that have to be made about the sample. One of the first considerations is to be clear on who or what will comprise the sample. For this to be achieved, unambiguous inclusion and exclusion criteria must be developed. This can be developed through reflection, discussion and by considering similar published research.

The type of study to be conducted, in terms of research approach or paradigm, will influence both the size of the sample and the method of selecting the sample. In the case of an experimental approach, a probability sampling method will be used with a reasonable sample size in each of the experimental and control groups, again guided by the experiences of similar studies. If relationships are sought but ethical or practical constraints prevent random allocation, then a quasi-experimental or ex post facto approach may be used.

In survey designs, the important decision is the extent to which there is a need to generalise further than the sample group. This will influence the choice between probability and non-probability sampling methods. Where probability sampling methods are required, a sampling frame of all possible candidates for the study is required. This should be as complete as possible to avoid bias.

In surveys that are more exploratory, and do not require generalisations to be made to the larger population, and for qualitative studies, non-probability methods can be chosen. These are far more flexible and simple, and do not require a sampling frame of individuals.

In terms of sample size, the approach used will dictate whether a large sample of near 100 or above will be required, or whether smaller numbers of 10 or even less will be adequate.

When writing up a research report, the researcher should clearly specify the details of the sample in the methods section. This should include the rationale behind the inclusion and exclusion criteria, the sampling approach, and the choice of sample size. Any changes to the sample size during the study should also be indicated along with an examination of the possible impact this may have had on the study outcomes.

CRITIQUING RESEARCH

In critiquing research, one of the first areas to consider is the extent to which the inclusion and exclusion criteria may reduce or increase bias. What is the rationale given by the researcher for the choice of criteria? Using your own professional judgement, do those included seem more or less representative as a result of the selection criteria?

A common error is for the researcher to generalise further than the sampling criteria would allow. For instance, statements may be made about all women in pregnancy or labour, when the sample consisted of only primigravida women, or excluded those of a certain age, social class or other social characteristics. Similarly, attempts may be made to generalise to all midwives when the study only included hospital-based midwives and excluded those working in community settings.

Was the appropriate sampling method used in the study? There should be a clear rationale for the choice of sampling method, and clear details concerning the process of selecting the sample. This should be examined carefully to ensure that the correct procedures are evident. For example, if the researcher says a random sample was used, can we be sure they do not mean a convenience sample. If it is truly a random sample there should be mention of a sampling frame and table of random numbers or other device.

The influence of sample size should also be assessed. Does the researcher justify the size of the sample selected? In an experimental design was there any problem with the number of individuals dropping out of the study (subject mortality) that may have affected the extent to which the groups were comparable at the end of the study?

If the researcher is using a qualitative design, we should expect small numbers and not criticise them for a small sample. However, we should still expect some detail on the sample characteristics so that we can judge whether they were in a position to provide information on the phenomena that forms the focus of the study. The more detail provided on the sample the more able we are to judge the extent to which the researcher has been rigorous in the way the study has been conducted.

KEY POINTS

- Research rarely collects data from a total target population. Usually, research is conducted on a sample taken as representative of a larger group. A sample can consist of people, objects or events.
- A sample should be defined in terms of inclusion and exclusion criteria.
- Sampling methods vary according to whether the study takes an experimental, survey or qualitative approach. Sampling methods, or strategies, can be divided into probability and non-probability methods.
- Probability sampling methods allow generalisations to be made from the findings to the larger target population. Other options under this heading include simple random sampling, systematic random sampling, stratified random sampling, proportionate random sampling and cluster sampling. In experimental designs, random allocation is more usual, which relates to how individuals are allocated to the experimental and control groups.
- Non-probability sampling methods include opportunity or convenience sampling, quota sampling, snowball sampling and purposive sampling. These are usually used in surveys and/or qualitative methods.

- Although non-probability sampling methods are weaker in design, as it is not possible to say whether the findings are generally applicable, they are easier to use. In the case of qualitative research, it is not the intention to generalise to a wider population, only to say that certain issues can be identified as relevant when considering a topic or issue.
- Sample size is influenced by the nature of the study, the availability of subjects, and factors such as response rate. Experimental studies may be modest in size ranging from 25 to 40 in each group, to quite large numbers such as 100 to 200 or considerably more in each group. Similarly, surveys can range from around 20 to several hundreds. Qualitative research can be anything from under 10 to more usually around 12 to 20. These numbers are only rough guidelines, and should not be interpreted as anything more.

REFERENCES

Burns, N., Grove, S., 2009. The Practice of Nursing Research: Appraisal, Synthesis, and Generation of Evidence, sixth ed. Saunders, St Louis.

Byrom, S., Downe, S., 2010. 'She sort of shines': midwives' accounts of 'good' midwifery and 'good' leadership. Midwifery 26 (1), 126–137.

Holloway, I., Wheeler, S., 2010. Qualitative Research for Nurses, third ed. Wiley-Blackwell, Chichester.

Huber, U., Sandall, J., 2009. A qualitative exploration of the creation of calm in a continuity of carer model of maternity care in London. Midwifery 25 (6), 613–621.

McDonald, S., Henderson, J., Faulkner, S., Evans, S., Hagan, R., 2010. Effect of an extended midwifery postnatal support programme on the duration of breast feeding: A randomised controlled trial. Midwifery 26 (1), 88–100.

Polit, D., Beck, C., 2008. Nursing Research: Generating and Assessing Evidence for Nursing Practice, eighth ed. Lippincott Williams and Wilkins, Philadelphia.

Procter, S., Allan, T., Lacey, A., 2010. Sampling. In: Gerrish, K., Lacey, A. (Eds.), The Research Process in Nursing, sixth ed. Wiley-Blackwell, Chichester.

Schmidt, N., Brown, J., 2009. Evidence-Based Practice for Nurses: Appraisal and Application of Research. Jones and Bartlett, Sudbury.

The challenge of the future

15

The last chapter of a novel usually reveals all, and brings the plot to a resolution. It often has a happy or at least intriguing ending, so that the reader puts down the book with a feeling of contentment, perhaps mixed with a tinge of regret that the characters will no longer be a feature of their life. Non-fiction books are not like that. The aim of this chapter is to emphasise that what has gone before in the previous chapters is only the beginning. This chapter challenges you to continue absorbing and applying the information in this book on an increasingly regular basis as part of your clinical practice. It will also encourage you to make a vital contribution to evidence-based practice by helping to establish a research culture in midwifery. This is the last chapter but it is not goodbye.

The future of maternity care is likely to be demanding as well as challenging for the midwife. For example, a report by the King's Fund (2008) identified the following changes that are likely to have future implications for maternity services:

- The number of births has risen since 2002 and is projected to increase.
- There is an increased number of older mothers, with higher rates of complication.
- There is more fertility treatment, leading to a higher rate of multiple births.
- There are more obese women, who are less fit for pregnancy.
- There are more women surviving serious childhood illness going on to have children, and needing extra care in pregnancy and childbirth.
- There is a rising rates of intervention in labour, in particular in rates of Caesarean section.
- An increasing social and ethnic diversity sometimes leads to communication difficulties and other social and clinical challenges in maternity care.

Such changes will require an even greater emphasis on an efficient midwifery service in order to cope with the complexity of demands. Despite successes with such developments as models of midwifery-led care (Hatem et al. 2009) there is still more work to be done in maintaining high levels of normality in women. The danger is that in stressful situations such as increasing demands

© 2011 Elsevier Ltd. All rights reserved.

and shortages of staff, workable solutions for reducing the problems can sometimes be rejected as a reaction to the situation (McKellar et al. 2009). So, although evidence-based practice offers practical ways of introducing improvements, the production and use of good-quality research may be seen as too demanding by those involved. In this situation, how can we build a culture that embraces evidence-based practice?

One option when looking at the future is to examine the past and previous aspirations for midwifery's future in research. This may provide a clue to how far we have come and what still needs to happen. Here is the '10 year wish list' for midwifery research made by Lavender et al. (2003: S22). See how many have come true.

- All midwives will have the confidence, ability, desire and opportunity to be involved in research.
- Access to appropriate resources in each clinical area, e.g. libraries, databases and research support staff, will be available.
- Multidisciplinary collaboration, which generates professional respect and equal status, will be encouraged. Multidimensional perspectives can only benefit the women and their families.
- External funding bodies will recognise the importance of midwifery research.
- Trusts will fund and support permanent midwifery research posts.
- Midwives will hold positions of high status to ensure midwifery research is a priority.
- Clinical and managerial leaders will all have research skills and the ability to support and facilitate and generate research in the clinical area.
- Dissemination of findings will be valued and midwives will be supported to attend appropriate forums.
- Local strategies will be developed to ensure the implementation and evaluation of research findings.

You do not always get everything you wish for, so we should acknowledge these as aspirations or directions in which we needed to go. Looking at the list, it is striking that many are now developing, but we are not there yet and the extent of successes of some of these will vary locally. None of the above has dropped completely off the wish list, although some progress has been made in most if not all of them. However, it is now time to consider where we set our sights for the next 10 years so that we can plan how we arrive at that destination. The remainder of this chapter will consider some of the themes where we need to focus attention.

CLOSING THE CREDIBILITY GAP BETWEEN PRODUCING AND USING RESEARCH

If we are to close the credibility gap between the amount of research evidence generated and the extent to which it is used in practice, all midwives need to share the same philosophy and emphasis on continually moving professional knowledge forward. To achieve this we must constantly challenge the basis for activities and seek new evidence to support clinical decision making. This will be demanding, as midwives have been regarded as fairly passive in their engagement with the evidence-based agenda (Lavender 2010). The use of information requires the generation of that knowledge so we need to increase the amount of new midwifery research. This book has cited large numbers midwifery research, which would suggest that midwifery does regularly produce research. So where is the problem? The answer is that although the amount of midwifery research has increased, it is still more of a trickle than a steady stream. There are still only a small number of midwives producing research. In other words, there is a lack of research capacity, that is, a shortage of midwives who are actively engaged in producing high-quality research.

The challenge for the future, then, is to answer the following questions:

- Why is there so little midwifery research produced on a regular basis?
- Why don't midwives make more use of the available research?
- How can we improve the situation?

WHY IS THERE SO LITTLE MIDWIFERY RESEARCH?

Just as in nursing, research in midwifery is a comparatively new phenomenon where techniques and skills of research are still being refined. Research role models are just beginning to emerge in the form of consultant nurses, and midwives working as full-time researchers, often in academic or research units. However, in the case of consultant midwives, their workload does not always allow them to pursue and promote the research aspect of their role and so inspire and encourage the number of midwifery researchers to expand. The conclusion is that at the moment there is a lack of midwives developing practical skills in carrying out research.

If more research is to be produced we must develop acceptable ways of acquiring high-level skills in research design, data gathering and data analysis. These do not come from assignments that require midwifery students to produce a literature review or design a research proposal. Although these activities develop useful skills, isolated from the experience of undertaking research they merely serve to produce a new research theory–practice gap.

How can we increase the opportunities for midwives to gain research skills? This could take a variety of forms. Schools of Midwifery need to provide courses and study programmes where these skills can be developed. These courses should balance the theory of research with engaging with research activity. This means there should be more 'hands on' and practical elements in the teaching, such as design workshops and data collection and analysis in a 'safe' and 'coached' environment.

There should also be opportunities for midwives to shadow midwifery researchers both in clinical areas and to gain secondments to research units where these exist. More midwifery research scholarships should also be considered for trained staff. It is beyond the scope of this chapter to explore all the problems of funding, but this is a crucial area that has to be developed if midwifery is to gain the same level of experience as other health professional groups.

WHY DON'T MIDWIVES MAKE MORE USE OF RESEARCH?

Care for women will stagnate unless we apply available evidence to practice, but before research can support practice it must first be accessed (Chapter 6), then critically evaluated (Chapter 5). Lavender (2010: 114) suggests that midwives fall into the following five categories when it comes to their use of the research literature:

- non-users,
- reluctant users,
- selective users,
- rigid users,
- thoughtful users.

Each of the first four groups is in some way problematic, and will have implications for the type of care provided. The non-user is unlikely to be open to change and so may be practicing in ways that could be outdated and dangerous. The reluctant user is likely to maintain old systems of care and only use research occasionally as a way of avoiding criticism. Selective users are likely to use research that supports their way of doing things and ignore research that disagrees with favoured methods. The rigid user will not adapt research recommendations flexibly to local situations even though they may vary considerably from conditions and contexts in which original studies were undertaken (Amelink-Verburg et al. 2010). The ideal goal would be to move all of the former closer to the final category of the 'thoughtful user', which Lavender (2010) characterises as a midwife who can identify relevant evidence and apply it to an individual woman in a particular context.

What are some of the main barriers to research implementation? If you consider your own clinical area, or those you have encountered as a student, what prevents a greater use of the available research that could improve care? Numerous studies both in the UK and the USA have identified barriers to applying research to practice, and these have been grouped by Gerrish (2010) under the following headings:

- *Barriers to do with the nature of the evidence*: This relates to the amount and quality of research available that either has not been generated, is poor in quality or not applicable to the context in which the practitioner wants to apply it.
- *Barriers to do with the way the evidence is communicated*: Problems with getting hold of some journals that contain relevant articles and the language in which they are written can make evaluation a problem for some clinicians.
- *Barriers to do with knowledge and skills of the individual nurse*: This relates to both the IT skills required in searching databases and accessing information, and to the skill of critically evaluating research reports.
- *Barriers to do with the organisation*: This relates not only to access problems in the clinical area and support in developing skills to evaluate the research, but also limitations on the power to effect or influence change as well as lack of support from key managers and leaders.

Together, these areas illustrate the many barriers facing midwifery that need to be surmounted if it is to be more research based. The relevance of these categories is that they form a diagnostic tool to identify the source of problems in a particular clinical area.

HOW CAN WE IMPROVE THE SITUATION?

It is easy to shrug shoulders and feel that the barriers to progress are insurmountable. However, the many places where research and evidence-based practice thrive demonstrate that change is possible. What is required is a strategy for achieving change. In terms of specific goals, although time is always identified as a major problem, we also need to develop a challenging approach to practice and embrace an evidence-friendly culture in the clinical setting. The starting point for this is a shared belief that research is needed to benefit practice. Our view of research should be broad, and avoid seeing it as synonymous with the randomised control trial (RCT). Certainly this is a demanding goal to achieve, but one that must be accomplished if a holistic approach to midwifery is to be maintained.

So far in its short life, evidence-based practice has focused on quantitative evidence. However, now there are signs that qualitative research is becoming a potential player in developing guidelines for practice. One example in nursing is a move to identify what patients value as important contributors to the quality of the care they receive. Hopkins (2010) suggests that nursing should develop patient-related outcome measures (PROMs) and that qualitative research highlighting patient experiences should help to construct meaningful quality outcome measures of care. This would allow practitioners to plan and improve experiences for those travelling through health care services. Midwifery has produced a large number of qualitative studies, as both share a person-centred, holistic perspective (Holloway and Wheeler 2010). These studies have illuminated the experiences, interpretations and meaning given by those involved in maternity care, and can be used to develop PROMs, or, more accurately, 'woman related outcome measures' (WROMs) in similar ways to that suggested by Hopkins (2010).

We also need to rethink our attitude towards change, and see it as a fundamental feature of the continued drive towards better care. Understandably, many midwives do not have a neutral attitude towards change. The past has seen many developments that have not made midwifery easier, or improved the quality of care given to women. This has led to scepticism and distrust towards change. Similarly, health professionals have traditionally felt very threatened by change and see suggestions for change as a personal attack on their clinical judgement. We need to find ways in which change can be discussed and examined positively, without it being seen as a personal threat or attack. This requires a more open systems view of change and an understanding of the complexity of forces involved in introducing change. This means that an additional skill required if midwifery is to progress is the art of change management.

A further need is for a greater political awareness within the profession of the influence of power in limiting women's access to the kind of service that best suits their needs. This is an under-represented theme in the research literature. Examples can be seen from countries such Southern Ireland (Keating and Fleming 2009) and Canada (Parry 2008) which have both produced examples of qualitative research focusing on women's use of midwifery services that reflect this political dimension of power, control and access to appropriately designed services.

15 DEVELOPING A DYNAMIC RESEARCH CULTURE IN MIDWIFERY

The way ahead lies in more midwives developing research skills, both in carrying out research and in developing skills in critically analysing published work. Firstly, under developing research skills, we should not expect every midwife to carry out research. Not everyone has the inclination, motivation, or availability of time to become involved in research. Yet someone needs to do it. We need more midwifery researchers producing high-quality research to inform practice.

How do we develop a research-producing culture? One useful development has been the number of midwives involved in audit. This is only a short step away from research. The two activities are very close, and should be carried out with the same attention to rigour. The similarities are such that the midwife proficient in audit has only to broaden the questions and develop an understanding of the thinking behind research to move closer to becoming a researcher. As audit draws in the main on quantitative approaches, it would be useful to extend the repertoire of skills by undertaking a research course, either as a stand-alone module, or as part of a higher degree course.

More midwives must be encouraged to carry out good research. Midwifery needs to develop a sound research base by firstly developing a research agenda of areas that need to be examined and then investigating these. At the same time midwives should participate in multidisciplinary research to ensure that midwifery also influences research by other professional groups (Amelink-Verburg et al. 2010). This kind of activity is the sign of a mature profession. It is not a case of taking midwives out of clinical practice; it is enhancing that practice through informed researchers.

This book has already attempted to provide an understanding of the ways in which midwives can become critical readers of research (Chapter 5). Although this is a useful quality for the individual, it becomes even more valuable where it contributes to a research culture. This means sharing the results of critiquing with others, firstly, on a small informal basis with colleagues who may also be developing this skill, and then with a larger group of midwives. This can be as part of a small research appreciation group, or as a journal club that provides the opportunity to reflect on practice and be open to change and ways of achieving it. The idea of journal clubs has been supported by Veeramah (2008) as a way of promoting the use of research findings in practice by keeping up to date with the latest research, and improving the quality of care provided. Critical reviews of the literature can also be undertaken by small groups of midwives as a basis for establishing clinical standards, or as a way of solving clinical problems or simply exploring new techniques and practices.

Both critiquing and reviewing the literature are high-level skills that are developed with guidance and practice. In carrying out these activities, it is also important to use professional knowledge, judgement and reflection as well as being creative in the use of the available work. However, do not expect to find the perfect answers to the problems facing you. It is often a case of skilfully applying knowledge from one area to suit the needs of a slightly different clinical setting whilst recognising the possible limitations that may be the inevitable consequence of this.

Evidence-based practice provides the ideal opportunity to develop a meaningful research culture in midwifery. This should not only improve the use of research, but also place it within the context of professional midwifery practice and the needs and wishes of women. However, this requires strong clinical leadership and proactive midwives uniting to decide on topics that could benefit from a clearer evidence base. This may result in a working group of staff to examine the literature and develop suitable guidelines that will later be audited. This provides the necessary stimulus to get started and develop applicable skills. This should then lead to those involved identifying further areas for investigation from their own experience and reflections on practice. Which topics could be examined? In nursing there has been a call for a focus on research into basic, or more appropriately, 'essential' nursing care and a move away from studies into areas of interest to areas of need (Cleary-Holdforth and Leufer 2009). This seems an excellent pattern to adopt in midwifery where those working in research should be encouraged to consider some of the key areas of midwifery to provide a better evidence base.

This section has put forward some simple suggestions for developing a more dynamic research culture in midwifery. We do have to remember the inevitability of barriers to change and that the best change may be in the form of a gradual evolution rather than a revolution. In other words, it is better to start in a modest way rather than have high aspirations dashed by a lack of overall support and commitment. It is better to start with a small group of enthusiasts and then work outwards, taking into account perhaps local initiatives and efforts to increase research capital within midwifery. These suggestions should be used to consolidate and extend the way we think about the midwife's role and developments for the future. An important aspect of this is to balance the science of research with the natural creativity and 'craft' of midwifery.

CONDUCTING RESEARCH

The starting point for research is to have a clear question that needs to be answered. The aim of this chapter has been to encourage midwives to think about their part in taking research forward, and one way is by carrying out research. This does not have to be elaborate, time consuming or costly. Small-scale projects can have equally useful ramifications for clinical practice, policy and resources. Unless individuals stop thinking about possibilities and take the step to participate in research, the 'tipping point' that provides the momentum for something meaningful to take off will not be reached (Gladwell 2001).

To carry out research successfully, it is important to have support from professional and managerial colleagues. You must possess a good level of research knowledge and be able to call upon an experienced researcher or research supervisor to provide guidance. It is important that the project remains yours and does not become something your research supervisor or adviser would really like to do themselves. In research, you also need a great deal of luck. There is never the perfect research project, and you must always expect the unexpected. It is a little like working with technology; if something can go wrong then it usually will. The compensation is that research is a truly exciting activity. Despite the accusation that researchers find only what they want to find, if you have designed your project rigorously and with the minimum of personal bias, there is no telling what you will find. And that's what makes it fun!

Once your study is complete, it must be communicated, firstly to managers who may have supported it and, where possible, to those who may have taken part, even if this takes the form of a one-page summary, to let them know that their participation contributed to something tangible. If the study was completed rigorously, then whether the results were positive or negative, a clear attempt should be made to disseminate it widely. This is supported by Amelink-Verburg et al. (2010) who encourage those who have completed research to be visible by publishing and presenting their work. This can be in the form of what Schmidt and Brown (2009) refer to as the 3 'P's of dissemination, namely:

- a conference poster,
- a conference paper,
- a journal article, i.e. publication.

Each has its own format and audience, and serves a different function. Poster presentations are a good introduction to research presentations, as they expose you to the minimum of intimidation. These depend on visual impact, and gaining the viewer's attention. First, try to attend a conference that has a wide variety of posters so that you can gain some good ideas. Do not forget to include your name and email address on the poster so people can get in touch with you for more information. It is also a good idea to provide a brief summary of the research that people can take away, but again include your name and contact details. For both conference and poster presentations, business cards will be extremely useful, and will save you writing down your email address in a hurry for people. Posters are an ideal way to 'sell' your research findings directly to those who are interested in them. As posters are so portable and have impact, they can also be used to great effect in the clinical area.

A conference paper requires verbal and visual presentation skills, good voice projection, enthusiasm and a willingness to share your work with a group. Powerpoint presentations can support the conference paper by emphasising key points and words and easy to assimilate tables that are neither too small to see nor too crowded with information. Many health organisations hold local conferences that are an ideal means of communicating your findings to a large and often mixed group of health professionals.

A journal article is one of the best ways to communicate your research to a wide audience. Journal articles differ depending on the journal, as each has its target audience and journal style. Do not submit to more than one journal at a time. It is acceptable to rework your article, once published, for another journal as long as it is not simply a rehash. Focus instead on a slightly different theme. Do not try to condense a whole dissertation or long assignment into a four thousand word or less article, just concentrate on two or three of the main themes. Make the article interesting by thinking of it from the reader's point of view.

If you are new to writing articles, seek the advice of someone who has already published. Co-authorship is also an alternative where you enlist the skills of someone with publishing experience, but always insist on your name going first.

The usual structure for conference papers, posters, or articles is as follows:

- Introduction to the topic (what was the problem?).
- What does the literature say about it?
- What was the research aim?
- How did you go about it (methods and sample)?
- What did you find (results)?
- What does it all mean (discussion)?
- What do you recommend?

Whichever medium is chosen, remember your audience, and the message you are communicating. Do not perpetuate the myth that research is written in gobbledygook by using over-elaborate 'scientific' language and research terms and concepts that require a great deal of prior knowledge from the reader. Where technical terms are used, make sure that their meaning is clear to the novice. Remember, you were there once, and the aim is to clarify not mystify.

CRITIQUING RESEARCH

Throughout this book emphasis has been placed on the skill of critiquing. This is a prerequisite for moving the culture of midwifery forward. Practice is needed in critiquing and each article will present its own challenges. Midwives, to use Lavender's (2010) phrase, should be the 'thoughtful user' of researcher. In other words, it is more than understanding research, it is about applying the literature carefully to the individual situation and woman. This was the original meaning of evidence-based practice when Sackett et al. (1996) described it as the 'judicious (well thought out) use of evidence', that is, it needs to be 'used with care'.

In this final chapter we should think not only of critiquing research but also of undertaking reviews of the literature (see Chapter 5) and implementing the findings where relevant. This might also mean ensuring that staff have the skills or are helped to acquire the skills indicated by the proposed change.

We also need to disseminate the critiques and reviews of the literature to contribute to a research culture. This will not be an easy task. Although evidence-based practice depends on all those in a clinical area agreeing standards, we may have to start small and develop important skills before we work effectively on the bigger picture. At a preliminary stage we should be satisfied with a small group of individuals who can share the same enthusiasm. We will not gain the support of everyone. A small successful 'journal club', or research interest group will be more satisfying and beneficial than a large group where only a small number attend, and you end up doing all the work.

Research folders containing articles accessible in the clinical area, and research notice boards are additional ways to disseminate information, providing they are regularly updated. Some invited speakers will also stimulate interest, but do not plan these for when most people are on holiday or when there is something else going on. A guest speaker and three people can be embarrassing and hard work. I know; I have been that guest speaker.

The final stage is research implementation, that is, the development of practice on the basis of firm evidence, often through clinical standards, guidelines or frameworks (Amelink-Verburg et al. 2010, Shallow 2010).

Despite the gains made since the introduction of evidence-based practice, evidence-based midwifery remains an uncomfortable place to be (Spiby and Munro 2010). However, change is always familiar territory, and midwives must reduce the evidence–practice gap. This is now down to you and your contribution to making maternity care woman-centred and firmly based on the philosophy of midwifery supported by the most appropriate evidence available.

KEY POINTS

- Midwifery research is on the point of entering a new era of maturity. The challenge is to increase the amount of quality research produced, critically evaluated and, where appropriate, implemented. The credibility gap between the amount of research produced and the amount put into practice must be reduced. Emphasis must be placed on developing a supportive midwifery research culture.
- More midwives need the practical skills of undertaking research. There is no shortage of clinical problems that need examining, and new developments that need evaluation. More encouragement is needed for midwives to develop these skills, and support given to undertake research, underpinned by an efficient system of funding.
- Once complete, midwifery research should be communicated by means of conference papers, posters and published articles. These should be seen as a crucial part of the research process and be clear, unambiguous and action orientated.
- One of the largest areas of deficit is the number of midwives who can critique research articles and produce critical reviews of the literature. When these activities are undertaken they should contribute to the wider research culture of the clinical area as clinical developments or clinical-effectiveness initiatives.
- The suggestions made in this chapter require someone to accept the challenge of the future. Let it be you.

REFERENCES

Amelink-Verburg, M., Herschderfer, K., Offerhaus, P., Buitendijk, S., 2010. The development of evidence based midwifery in the Netherlands: the journey from midwifery knowledge to midwifery research to midwifery standards of practice. In: Spiby, H., Munro, J. (Eds.), Evidence-Based Midwifery: Applications in Context. Wiley-Blackwell, Chichester.

Cleary-Holdforth, J., Leufer, T., 2009. Evidence-based practice: Sowing the seeds for success. Nurse Educ. Pract. 9 (5), 285–287.

Gerrish, K., 2010. Evidence-based practice. In: Gerrish, K., Lacey, A. (Eds.), The Research Process in Nursing, sixth ed. Wiley-Blackwell, Chichester.

Gladwell, M., 2001. The Tipping Point: How Little Things Can Make A Big Difference. Abacus, London.

Hatem, M., Sandall, J., Devane, D., Soltani, H., Gates, S. 2009. Midwife-led versus other models of care for childbearing women (Review). The Cochrane Collaboration, Published by JohnWiley & Sons. Available: http://apps.who.int/rhl/reviews/CD004667.pdf (accessed 23.05.10.).

Holloway, I., Wheeler, S., 2010. Qualitative Research for Nurses, third ed. Wiley-Blackwell, Chichester.

Hopkins, A., 2010. Using qualitative research to improve tissue viability care. Nurs. Stand. 24 (32), 64–67.

Keating, A., Fleming, V., 2009. Midwives' experiences of facilitating normal birth in an obstetric-led unit: a feminist perspective. Midwifery 25 (5), 518–527.

King's Fund, 2008. Safe Births: Everybody's Business. An Independent Enquiry into the Safety of Maternity Services in England. King's Fund, London.

Lavender, T., 2010. Is there enough evidence to meet the expectations of a changing midwifery agenda? In: Spiby, H., Munro, J. (Eds.), Evidence-Based Midwifery: Applications in Context. Wiley-Blackwell, Chichester.

Lavender, T., Briscoe, L., Baker, L., 2003. The evolution and destiny of midwifery research. British Journal of Midwifery 11 (10), S18–S22.

McKellar, L., Pincombe, J., Henderson, A., 2009. Encountering the culture of midwifery practice on the postnatal ward during Action Research: An impediment to change. Women Birth 22, 112–118.

Parry, D., 2008. 'We wanted a birth experience, not a medical experience'. Exploring Canadian women's use of midwifery. Health Care Women Int. 29 (8), 784–806.

Sackett, D., Rosenberg, W., Gray, J., Haynes, R., Richardson, W., 1996. Evidence based medicine, what it is and what it isn't. Br. Med. J. 312, 71–72.

Schmidt, N., Brown, J., 2009. Evidence-Based Practice for Nurses: Appraisal and Application of Research. Jones and Bartlett, Sudbury.

Shallow, H., 2010. Guidelines and the consultant midwife: the challenges of the interdisciplinary guideline group. In: Spiby, H., Munro, J. (Eds.), Evidence-Based Midwifery: Applications in Context. Wiley-Blackwell, Chichester.

Spiby, H., Munro, J., 2010. Evidence based midwifery: current status and future priorities. In: Spiby Hand Munro, J.(Ed.), Evidence-Based Midwifery: Applications in Context. Wiley-Blackwell, Chichester.

Veeramah, 2008. Exploring strategies for promoting the use of research findings in practice. Br. J. Nurs. 17 (7), 466–471.

GLOSSARY OF COMMON RESEARCH TERMS

Abstract: Published reports and dissertations usually begin with an abstract. This is a one or more paragraphs giving a brief, but succinct overview of the study. If you read this, you should be able to establish if the study is relevant to your.

Accidental sampling/sample: See *Convenience sampling*.

Action research: A research design that involved the introduction and evaluation of change. There is no control group, which makes generalisations difficult. However, something is introduced which might make a positive difference to the setting. Its advantage is that it involves those in this setting deciding what should take place and how. It has a great potential in midwifery practice, but is probably underutilised.

After-only design: Form of experimental design where there is only one measurement taken following the introduction of an intervention. This has the advantage of not building on previous exposure to information or measurements. However, the disadvantage is that there is no baseline available to know if there has been any improvement from a previous level. An alternative is the pre-test post-test design where measurements are made both before and after the intervention.

Alternative hypothesis: Although this is known as the alternative, it is the form that is more familiar than its opposite, the null-hypothesis, which suggests there is no difference between the groups under study. The alternative hypothesis, sometimes called the scientific hypothesis, is the automatic opposite of the null-hypothesis and predicts that there is a difference between the groups that is unlikely to have happened by chance.

ANCOVA: Abbreviation of **AN**alysis of **COVA**riance. This is a statistical procedure used to test mean differences among groups on a dependent variable and tries to ensure that other variables (covariates) are not influencing the apparent relationship.

ANOVA: Similar to the above and stands for **AN**alysis **O**f **VA**riance. This tests the mean difference between three or more groups and compares how much variability there is within the groups as well as between them.

Anonymity: An essential principle of ethics that protects the identity of individuals who have taken part in a study. Achieved by avoiding use of personal names or identifying details about the individual or setting.

Applied research: Research that seeks to solve a practical problem rather than simply add to our knowledge on a topic or concept.

Attention factor: Explanation for changes in behaviour due to participants reacting to being in a study. See also: *Hawthorn effect*.

Audit trail: In qualitative research the detail that indicates the way the researcher moved from individual quotes, or observations, to key categories used to make sense of the findings. This contributes to the credibility of the research.

Auditability: In qualitative research, the judgement that the researcher has provided sufficient detail to allow the reader to follow an audit trial and confirm the researcher's conclusions.

© 2011 Elsevier Ltd. All rights reserved.

Authenticity: Part of the criteria for assessing the soundness of qualitative research. It demonstrates what attempts were made to check the accuracy of the findings, e.g. member's check where participants confirm the accuracy of what was recorded. A further method is the use of 'thick' or rich descriptions of the way in which the study was conducted and the environments and incidents encountered. These should allow readers to feel almost as though they are there.

Autonomous or Autonomy: This means 'self-governing' and relates to the basic ethical principles of the right of individuals to make decisions about themselves and whether to take part in a study.

Back chaining: In searching or sourcing the literature, a method of finding further studies by consulting the references in a particular publication. See also: *forward chaining*.

Bar graph: A way of illustrating the results of quantitative research in the form of blocks which help the reader to see differences between variables and groups. They differ from histograms, as bar graphs have a space between each bar, since the data are discrete, such as primigravida and multigravida, and not continuous data such as height or weight.

Baseline measurements: These are measurements made before a change or intervention takes place. This acts as a comparison for later measurements. Used in experimental studies as part of the 'before' measurement.

Basic research: The opposite of applied research. The purpose is to add to knowledge or theory on a topic or concept.

Before and after designs: A type of experimental design, also known as a pre-test post-test design, where measurements are taken before an intervention and after. This has the advantage of establishing changes from a baseline measure. In some situations, however, it can be a disadvantage as people are sensitised to issues or abilities that may influence the performance on the 'after' part of the measurement. An alternative is the after-only design.

Beneficence: In ethics, relates to the principle of doing only good and avoiding harm. This principle ensures that the researcher considers how the study will be of benefit.

Blinding: Also called '**masking**'. The procedure involved in hiding from those involved in a randomised control trial (RCT) who is receiving which intervention. It is used to reduce the possibility that subjects will behave differently if they believe they are receiving a beneficial treatment. A single-blind study is where the subjects are unaware of which intervention they are receiving, and double-blind is where both the subjects and those measuring outcomes or providing care are unaware of an individual's group membership. This is taken as an element of rigour in RCTs and is sometimes a criterion for the inclusion of studies in a systematic review of the literature. Blinding is not possible in all interventions (e.g. episiotomies) when an intervention is clearly apparent.

Blind review: This does not relate to the conduct of a study, but to the process of publication. It is a system whereby those asked to evaluate the suitability of an article for publication are not given the names of the authors. This reduces the accusation that only certain people's work appears in print. It is designed to ensure fair publishing opportunities where work is chosen on merit, not on the name of the author.

Bias: Anything that distorts or affects the study in a way that will alter or influence the accuracy of the findings. Usually relates to an untypical or unrepresentative sample but can relate to other elements. It is not always easy to spot bias: you need to ask whether there is anything about the way the study was conducted that could have had an adverse influence on the accuracy of the findings.

Bimodal distribution: A statistical description of the distribution of a variable where the data indicate there are two values that occur with equal frequency. Plotted on a graph, a bimodal distribution would be indicated by two peaks.

Bracketing: In qualitative research, researchers are encouraged to identify their own experiences or expectations that may influence their preconceived ideas about the study, and put aside or 'bracket' these so that they do not unduly influence interpretations of the findings. There is some controversy over the extent to which this is possible to achieve.

Case study: This is an in-depth study of a single individual or location, such as a clinical area, used to develop insights. The generalisability of the results is low as it depends on how representative the individual or location is of their kind.

Causal relationship: The objective of experimental designs is to establish evidence of a causal relationship between an independent variable (the cause) and a dependent variable (the effect). It is confirmed by the statistical relationship between the two variables.

Cell: Tables displaying the results of research are often divided into a number of segments or boxes. These are referred to as cells. One of the most frequently encountered tables is the 2×2 table that has four cells, e.g. male, female, yes and no.

Chi-squared test (χ^2): (Pronounced 'ki-squared'): In statistics, a non-parametric test that seeks to establish if the difference between the observed results of a categorical variable (e.g. male, female) is statistically different from the expected value, and is unlikely to have happened by chance.

CINAHL: An abbreviation for the database Cumulative Index Nursing and Allied Health Literature. Used in the process of reviewing the literature.

Clinical trial: Research approach that tests the effectiveness of a particular clinical intervention in an experimental design. Statistical analysis is used to establish the extent to which differences between treatments could be due to chance factors.

Closed questions: Used in questionnaires or interviews where the respondent is only provided with certain options from which to choose. This makes analysis an easy counting job but may not accurately represent the respondent's true answer.

Coding: Method of analysing qualitative data where an identifying name or category heading is given to recurring items or themes running through the findings.

Cohort: In sampling, a total group from whom data are collected.

Concept definition: The meaning or definition of a concept used by the researcher in the study. This is stated to clarify the meaning and avoid confusion with competing definitions.

Confirmability: Used in qualitative research as part of ensuring the researcher has demonstrated that the findings are accurate, genuine, and a true representation of the processes involved. If the researcher has met the criteria of *auditability*, *credibility*, and *fittingness*, then confirmability is achieved.

Confounding variable: A variable, often in an experimental study, that may influence (confound or cloud) the outcome and get in the way of a clear explanation of the results.

Consent form: Used as part of ethical principles to ensure the researcher can demonstrate that informed consent has been given. Those taking part in the study, or someone acting on their behalf if this is not possible, should sign this. A witness to the signature who is not a health professional may also be required.

Constructivist research: Another term for qualitative research based on the belief that people construct their reality on the basis on their interpretation and meaning they give to important elements in their life. The role of the qualitative researcher is to map the way constructions are achieved by individuals.

Continuous data: A form of data where the measurements flow along a single scale incrementally, such as height, blood pressure, and age. The opposite is discrete data, where items fall into one category or another and do not flow along a numeric scale, e.g. male, female.

Control: An essential feature of experimental design where the researcher has control over the design, particularly in regard to variables that might influence the findings of the study.

Control group: In an experimental design, the subjects who receive the usual treatment, or placebo, and not the intervention or form of the independent variable being tested. The results of measurements from the control group are compared with those of an *experimental group* to establish the existence of a cause-and-effect relationship.

Constant comparative method: In qualitative research, this is a method of analysing the data where comparisons are made with previously noted items or categories to ensure consistency in the method of analysis.

Convenience sampling: Also called **opportunity or accidental sampling**. A non-probability sampling method that uses those who are in the right place at the right time, and are willing to participate in a study. The limitation is there is little to guarantee they are representative of the total group. However, it is a cheap, quick way of collecting data, and the findings may not be that dissimilar from more expensive probability methods.

Correlation studies: The aim of these is to reveal a clear pattern of association. It does not imply a cause-and-effect relationship, only that there is a consistent pattern between two variables. An example would be a correlation between breastfeeding mothers and social class. Social class does not cause women to breastfeed; it is merely a pattern or association that is seen to exist between the two. Although the pattern may be reasonably stable, it does not happen in all cases.

Correlation: A statistical technique that searches for a relationship between two variables in a study. A positive correlation means that as one variable increases, so does the other (e.g. height and weight); a negative correlation is where as one variable goes up, the other goes down (e.g. outdoor temperature and weight of clothing). The strength of a correlation is indicated by a *correlation coefficient*, which indicates how certain we can be that a clear pattern exists.

Covert observation: Where those in an observation study are unaware they are being observed. The opposite is overt observation where observation is carried out as a visible activity. Covert observations can raise ethical concerns, as informed consent may not have been given.

Credibility: Used in qualitative research to ensure that the findings are a true representation of what was said, seen or heard. One method of achieving this is to give informants transcripts of interviews or conversations to confirm as accurate. This is called a *member's check*.

Critique: A balanced assessment of a research study that considers not only the findings but also how it was conducted and its strengths and limitations.

Cross-sectional study: A survey that looks at a situation at one point in time by including different aspects of one group rather than following the same group over time (a longitudinal study), e.g. women at different points of pregnancy. This is more cost effective than a longitudinal study, but may come up with different findings than following the same group through time.

Crossover design study: Form of experimental design where a group receives firstly one intervention, is measured, and then receives a second intervention and is re-measured. This can be done with a single group, or more than one group. Individuals receive both interventions and act as their own control. The biggest problem is the carry-over effect, where the benefits of the first intervention may affect the evaluation of the second. Interventions are frequently randomly allocated to individuals to reduce this problem.

Cross-tabulation: One form of presenting a table of results where one variable, such as age, is broken down by another variable, e.g. parity.

Cultural strangeness: Technique used in qualitative research, especially ethnographic research, where researchers attempt to distance themselves from a familiar environment in order to see things through a stranger's eyes. The aim is to question taken-for-granted assumptions and activities.

Data: Information collected in a study.

Data saturation: See *Saturation*.

Deductive reasoning: This is a method of analysis that starts from general theories or propositions and then examines the specific results that may support these general statements. This approach characterises quantitative research, particularly experimental designs.

Dependability: Part of the criteria used to assess the authenticity of qualitative research. The researcher must demonstrate that the findings are credible through such mechanisms as prolonged and in-depth data gathering. If *credibility* is established, then dependability is said to have been achieved.

Dependent variable: In experimental design, the variable that forms the outcome measured in the study, or the 'effect'. The independent variable is the presumed 'cause'. So in a study examining the relationship between information-giving and feelings of control during a birth, the feelings of control during the birth would be the dependent variable or effect, and the information would be the independent variable, or cause.

Descriptive research: A research approach that seeks to paint a picture of a situation either in numbers, as in quantitative research, or words, as in qualitative research.

Descriptive statistics: One of the two main forms of statistical analysis that attempts to describe a situation in numbers. The second main form of statistics is *inferential statistics* that allow inferences to be made about the wider population from which the sample is taken.

Design: This is the plan of action followed by the researcher to achieve the goals of the research, e.g. survey design, experimental design.

Directional hypothesis: Also called the research hypothesis, where a clear prediction is made of the expected outcome between two groups in an experimental setting. This form of hypothesis is indicated by the use of such terms as 'greater than', 'smaller than', or 'more often than', in relation to the measurements between the experimental and control groups. Other forms of hypotheses include *non-directional*, and *null-hypothesis*.

Discrete data: Also called discontinuous data. A form of data where the measurements fall into clearly different categories, such as male and female. The opposite is continuous data where the measurements flow from one value to another on one scale incrementally, such as height, blood pressure, age.

Emic perspective: In qualitative research, this looks at things from the perspective of those experiencing it, using their own words. The opposite is the *etic* perspective, that is, the outsider or researcher's perspective, found in quantitative research.

Empirical evidence: The collection of data in the real world involving the senses of sight, touch and hearing, rather than through assumption or abstract development of an argument. Health service research is largely empirical. Empirical evidence is concrete information that has been gathered in the real world to answer a specific question.

Ethics: A code of research practices and principles considered correct. When planning research involving human subjects, the researcher must consider ethical principles including informed consent, anonymity, an estimation of any possible harm, and justice, that is, treating everyone fairly. These provide high-quality research and are part of research governance.

Etic: In qualitative research, the perspective of the researcher, or outsider. The opposite is the *emic* perspective, which is the insider view of things, in their own words.

Ethnography: A type of qualitative research that attempts to uncover the social world of a cultural group, clients, or health staff, from the perspective of those in the situation. It has its roots in anthropology and uses observation and interviews over a reasonable time period.

Evidence-based practice: A philosophy of basing clinical activity on sound evidence. Research, particularly in the form of randomised control trials, is a highly regarded source of such evidence. It should also take account of professional consensus of opinion and client acceptance. The aim is to follow best practice for each person receiving health care support.

Experimental design: A classic approach to research that aims to establish cause-and-effect relationships. It usually consists of two groups where an independent variable in the form of an intervention is contrasted with either usual procedures or a placebo. Accurate measurements are made of the dependent variable to establish statistically if any changes could have happened by chance, or whether the changes are due to the independent variable.

Experimental group: In an experimental design, those who receive the independent variable or intervention form the experimental group. The results are compared with a *control group*.

Experimental intervention: This is the form of the independent variable introduced into the experimental group in experimental design and not to those in the control group. It is this that is presumed to be the 'cause' in the cause-and-effect relationship that is the subject of the experiment.

Ex post facto: A research approach used where an experimental approach involving manipulation of the independent variable by the researcher is not possible. It consists of examining groups where the independent variable is already present in those forming one of the groups, e.g. smoking. Ex post facto literally means 'after the fact'. As it lacks manipulation and control, it is not as strong at indicating causal relationships as the experimental design, as the findings may be explained by other factors.

Face validity: A 'face value' judgement, often made by an expert, on the likelihood that a method of measurement will produce accurate results. Frequently used in relation to questionnaires and assessment scales.

Feminist research: A research approach that highlights the disadvantages and unsatisfactory situations facing women because they are women, with the intention of improving the situation.

Fieldwork: In qualitative research, data collection that takes place in the natural environment or setting in which those involved in the study are usually found. This is usually carried out for long periods of time in order to observe this group under a range of circumstances. It is the opposite of 'laboratory research' in quantitative research, which is an artificially constructed or controlled environment.

Fieldwork notes/diary: Part of data collection in qualitative research. These describe the details and personal thoughts kept by the researcher whilst engaged in a study and will be used as part of the study findings.

Findings: Often used as the qualitative equivalent to the quantitative term 'results', meaning the product of data gathering and analysis.

Fittingness: Used in qualitative research to indicate that the findings of the study may well apply to other situations but not in the exact way indicated by the term generalisability.

Fixed alternative questions: In questionnaire design, where respondents are given a list of alternatives from which to choose. The opposite is open questions.

Focus groups: Interview design that uses a small group of individuals to talk about their experiences, feelings or views.

Focused interviews: Where the interviewer uses a flexible and informal approach that centres on a broad list of topics or subject headings with a respondent.

Follow-up study: Used to return to respondents after an initial study to discover any changes or outcomes that have developed. This is a separate study from a previous one and not the same as a 'before and after' study.

Forced choice: See *Fixed alternative questions*.

Forward chaining: Similar to *back chaining* but instead of using one article's references to seek previous studies, it entails the identification of relevant articles in databases where the option 'cited by' is offered. This will take the searcher forward in time to more recent articles that have drawn on or made reference to a previous study.

Frequency distribution: In descriptive statistical presentations, the numbers falling into each of the categories used in the analysis of a question. Often shown in a table.

Gatekeeper: In qualitative research, used to refer to those in a setting who can control or limit the researcher's access to subjects, settings or events.

Generalisability: In quantitative research, the ability to apply the results of a study to similar situations. This is one of the aims of the quantitative research.

Grounded theory: A type of qualitative research where the aim is to produce an explanation or theory that is 'grounded' in the findings and arises inductively through the researcher's interpretation and analysis. Developed by two Americans, Barny Glaser and Anselm Strauss.

Hawthorne effect: Where the behaviour of individuals in a study may be influenced by the knowledge of their involvement or participation in a study. Similar to the placebo effect, this is an attention factor that is a threat to the validity of a study. The name is taken from an American study on worker motivation set in the Hawthorne electrical plant in Chicago.

Histogram: Line drawing used to display numeric results in the shape of a series of blocks. Histograms differ from bar graphs in that the blocks touch, as they use continuous rather than discrete data.

Historical research: A research design that looks systematically at past situations or problems, using historical records, objects, diaries and verbal or visual accounts produced by those who witnessed them.

Hypothesis: In experimental designs, this is the researcher's prediction of what they might find if the theory being tested can be supported. It outlines the relationship between the independent and dependent variables in the study. It can take a number of different forms such as directional, non-directional and 'null'.

Inclusion and exclusion criteria: In sampling, the characteristics that help to identify those who qualify to take part in the study (inclusion criteria) and those who may introduce bias and be unrepresentative, or who may be put at risk by participation (exclusion criteria).

Independent variable: In experimental research, this is the cause or intervention that is believed to influence an outcome or dependent variable.

Inductive reasoning or approach: This form of analysis starts with a group of observations or data that are used to formulate general principles that might explain the patterns or relationships apparent in the findings. This form of reasoning is a feature of qualitative research. It is the opposite of *deductive reasoning*, which starts with general principles, and then examines the data to confirm the explanation.

Inferential statistics: One of the two main categories of statistical analysis that use the numerical results of a study as the basis of inferences to a wider group. The second main form of statistics is *descriptive statistics*, which provides a numeric picture of a situation found in a study.

Informant: In qualitative research, the name given to the sample who provide information relevant to the aim of the study.

Informed consent: Also called *valid consent*. An ethical requirement to gain permission from an individual invited to take part in research, based on a full understanding of what will happen, possible advantages and disadvantages, and other relevant details. It is expected that this should be gained in writing.

Institutional review board (IRB): The American equivalent of a local research ethics committee (LREC). Its role is to provide ethical approval for studies.

Instrument: The tool used to collect data in a study such as a questionnaire or assessment scale.

Internal validity: The ability of the research design to measure the true effect of the intervention rather than the effect of influences outside the study.

Inter-rater reliability: The extent to which more than one data collector in a study assesses the same outcome, situation or result in an identical way.

Interval measurement: Level of measurement that produces numerical values. Differs from the higher category of ratio level in that it does not have an absolute zero.

Interview: Method of collecting data through face-to-face, telephone or interactive method (e.g. on-line). Can be on a one-to-one or focus group basis. Interviews vary in structure and depth.

Interview guide: Used in in-depth interviews as a way of providing a broad structure and direction. Takes the form of loosely formed questions, topics or subjects that can be referred to in a flexible way. Differs from an interview schedule that is more structured and fixed.

Interview schedule: Fixed list of questions similar to a questionnaire, used in interviews to produced standardised results. Differs from interview guide, which is more flexible.

Item: In a Likert scale, used to describe a statement to which the respondent may chose options ranging from 'strongly agree' or to 'strongly disagree'.

Judgemental sample: More commonly known as a purposive sample. This is a non-probability sampling strategy where those in the study are picked on the basis of the researcher's knowledge of their characteristics that will contribute to a balanced or representative sample.

Justice: The ethical principle that all those involved in research should be treated fairly and equally as human beings.

Key informant: In qualitative research, someone who has a special position in the setting or who has valuable information. Key informants provide the researcher with major insights or details crucial to the study.

Key word: In reviewing the literature, this is the word(s) entered into the database in order to discover what has been published under the topic investigated. Care is needed, as words commonly used may not be the same as those under which suitable articles are stored. American spellings can also be problematic.

Levels of measurement: A categorisation of the different properties of numbers. Includes nominal, ordinal, interval and ratio levels. These play an important part in determining the appropriate statistical tests that may be used with the data collected.

Level of significance: The 'p' or probability level in a study that indicates the extent to which the results could have happened by chance. The minimum level is usually set at '$p < 0.05$' which means that, statistically, there is less than five in a hundred chance of being wrong if the researcher maintained there was a relationship between the independent and dependent variables in the study.

Likert scale: A method of measuring opinion or attitude by asking respondents to 'strongly agree' to 'strongly disagree' with a list of statements or 'items' in an interview or questionnaire. Usually a five-point scale, this is named after the American Rensis Likert who developed the technique and so is spelt with a capital 'L'.

Limitations: All studies have their weaknesses. The researcher should identify those that may affect the outcome of the study and the interpretation of the results. This is usually found at the start of the discussion section.

Literature review: An essential aspect of research studies where researchers place their study within the context of what is already known about the topic and the recent research that has been conducted. This should be critical in nature, and not simply a summary of previous work. Reviews of the literature, especially in their more systematic form, also play an important role in evidence-based practice and in producing standards for audit.

Lived experience: In phenomenological research, an attempt to understand a situation or health condition through the eyes of those experiencing it, so we can gain insights and understanding.

Longitudinal study: A type of research that follows a group of individuals over a long period of time to gain an understanding or measurement of any long-term changes, experiences or effects of a variable. Can take the form of a *panel study* where the same people are followed over time, or a *trend study* where different people from the same population are included at different points of time. The time period may range from weeks or months to years.

Manipulation: A feature of experimental design where the researcher introduces a change in the situation or to the subjects in the study. This is usually the introduction of the independent variable, or intervention.

Matching: A method of sampling in experimental design where individuals are matched by the researcher in terms of key characteristics that may have an undue influence or confounding effect on the study outcome. The aim is to divide those with possible confounding attributes such as age, sex, parity equally between the different study groups so that the groups can be compared fairly. This reduces the effect of the confounding characteristic on the outcome, as it will affect each group equally.

Methodology or method: The overall design followed by researchers in carrying out their research, as in *survey method*, or *experimental method*. Each method will follow certain principles and set procedures. In everyday use, it is used as a heading in research reports under which the details of how the research was conducted are presented for scrutiny.

Maturation: One of the threats to the validity of an experimental design, where the outcome could be influenced by changes to the individual, either physically or mentally, over the course of the measurement period.

Mean: The statistical term for an average. It relates to what is typical in the group and is part of a series of measures called *measures of central tendency*.

Measure of central tendency: A statistical term for the result of a procedure that attempts to establish a typical single value from a set of numbers. We usually talk about an average, but there are three such measures: *mean, mode* and *median*. Each of these can produce a very different result because of the way in which they are calculated.

Median: A measure of central tendency or 'average' in a set of results that identifies the value of a number which is midway along a set of values put in order from smallest to largest. Fifty per cent of the values will be above that number and 50% below it. It is a stable measurement and is not unduly influenced by numbers that may be untypically large or small in the set.

MEDLINE: A database of medical journal articles, often accessed on-line.

Member's check: In qualitative research, the process of increasing credibility by getting those who provided data to check what has been written for accuracy.

Meta-analysis: A method of combining the results of a number of studies on the same topic, carried out in similar ways, in order to increase the total size of the study sample. If successful, this can increase the accuracy of the statistical procedures carried out on the data, and so increase the value of the prediction based on the combined outcomes. There are many difficulties in this procedure due to hidden variations and biases in the way different studies have been conducted.

Mode: A measure of central tendency or 'average' that identifies the value of the unit that appears most often in a set of numbers. It is not a good indicator of what is typical in a set of numbers. If two numbers appear in a set the same number of times they form a *bi-modal distribution*. If several numbers appear the same number of times, it is known as a *multi-modal distribution*.

Moderator: Term for a researcher facilitating a focus group. This is a highly skilled role.

Mortality: See *Study mortality*.

Naturalistic approach or paradigm: Used as an alternative description for qualitative research methods, where there is no attempt to control or manipulate, and the study takes places in a normal or natural setting rather than a carefully controlled laboratory setting. It represents a philosophical approach to thinking about the natural world and how it should be studied.

Nominal data: This is the most basic of the levels of measurement and relates to numbers that do not have a value in relation to quantity, but merely label a category with a number, e.g. primigravida = 1, multigravida = 2. It is not possible to carry out statistical procedures on nominal data apart from producing a frequency distribution, that is, how many were in each group.

Non-directional hypothesis: Here, a clear prediction is not made of the expected outcome between two groups in an experimental setting, only that a difference will be found. Unlike directional hypotheses that use such terms as 'greater than', 'smaller than' or 'more often than' in relation to the outcomes between the experimental and control group, non-directional hypotheses merely say there will be a difference. The nature of the difference and in which group it will be found is not stated.

Non-equivalent experimental designs: This indicates that those in a study have not been randomly allocated to the experimental or control group. This means that it is not possible to be certain that any differences are purely due to the independent variable; differences between those in the two groups could have influenced the outcome.

Non-experimental design: A study where the researcher does not introduce a variable and is not looking for a cause and effect relationship. It should not be inferred that research in this category is less worthy than experimental research, only that the intentions are different.

Non-maleficence: The ethical principle to do no harm in a study. This is one of the most powerful principles of ethical considerations.

Non-parametric statistics: A collection of statistical techniques to establish the likelihood of relationships amongst data that do not require the strict criteria of parametric statistics. This makes them easier to apply but the results are not as widely accepted or as accurate as those in the parametric category.

Non-probability sampling methods: A collection of frequently used methods of selecting the sample in a study that includes opportunity/accidental, quota and purposive sampling strategies. It is not possible to say with any certainty how typical those selected are of the larger population using any of these methods. Their advantage is that they are relatively easy to use.

Non-significant result: This does not mean that the results of the research are not important; it means that in the case of a randomised control trial the 'p value' is too large to rule out the element of chance and therefore the null-hypothesis must be accepted. In other words, there was no real difference between the results of the groups involved.

Normal distribution: This relates to a statistical pattern of the distribution of some variables such as height and blood pressure. If data on these variables were plotted on a graph for a sample group, they should produce a bell shaped curve where most people are close to the mean, and others are in equal proportion on either side of the mean. In a normal distribution the mean, mode and median all have the same value and graphically would be a single line dropping down from the apex of the frequency curve. A normal distribution allows the use of parametric statistical tests, making this an important statistical concept.

Null-hypothesis: This is the hypothesis of no difference, that is, it predicts that there will be no statistically significant differences between the outcome measures for the groups in the study. It is also called the statistical hypothesis. It is expressed in this way because it is easier to reject the null-hypothesis than it is to accept its opposite, the research hypothesis, which predicts a real difference between the results of the groups in the study. If the null-hypothesis is rejected, it leads to the automatic acceptance of the research or directional hypothesis.

Nuremberg code: Ethical principles applied to experimental research on humans. Designed to prevent inappropriate and dangerous research by protecting those involved, it is based on 10 principles, including informed consent.

Observation: Method of collecting research data through visible means, using either the eye or a camera. This can be structured in the form of quantitative checklists, or unstructured, in the form of qualitative participant or non-participant observation.

Observer drift: Loss of concentration by the researcher in observation studies where observations are carried out over extended period. Shorter periods or time sampling may be a solution.

One-tailed hypothesis: Also called a directional hypothesis, this predicts a difference between two groups in the study and is indicated by the use of such words as 'more than' or 'less than'.

Open coding: The method of qualitative analysis where codes, or 'category headings' are given to the categories identified in the data.

Open (ended) questions: In questionnaire or interview designs, where respondents are encouraged to provide a response in their own words rather than choosing from a list of choices.

Operational definition: The way in which the researcher intends to measure or 'make operational' the variables under study.

Opportunity sampling: See *Convenience sampling*.

Ordinal level of measurement: The category that follows nominal data. Here, the numbers used relate to the position or order of the items along a simple measuring scale (first, second, etc.). As with nominal data, there are severe restrictions on the statistical procedures that can be carried out on them. Examples include Likert scales that go in order from 'strongly disagree' to 'strongly agree'.

Outliers: In a set of numeric measures, these are the values at the extreme ends of a distribution that are not necessarily typical of the others in the set, e.g. those untypically old or young in a group.

Overt observation: Where the research activities of an observer are clearly visible and known by those involved to be taking place. The opposite is covert observation, where those in the setting do not know they are being observed.

'P' value: This is the indicator that the researcher has statistically tested the results, particularly in randomised control trials, to establish the 'probability' that the differences could be due to chance, and not the intervention. The most common values used to indicate that the results are unlikely to have happened by chance are, in increasing size of certainty that the results are real differences, $p < 0.05$, 0.01 and 0.001.

Panel study: This kind of longitudinal study takes the form of a survey where the same people are approached for information at two or more points over time. This provides information on how people, variables or experiences change over time.

Paradigm: A distinct way of looking at the world around us that colours all aspects of our understanding; it is a 'world view'. An example is the way obstetrics and medicine have been characterised as illustrating a different paradigm or view of the world compared to midwifery and nursing.

Participant observer: Where the researcher observes whilst carrying out similar activities in the setting as those being observed.

Phenomenology: A qualitative approach that seeks to uncover the 'lived experience' of people in a particular setting or with a particular health condition or status, e.g. the lived experience of parenting triplets.

Physiological measurement: A precise way of measuring some physiological factor or outcome, e.g. temperature or blood pressure.

Pilot study: A small-scale test to ensure that the tool of data collection is reliable and that there are no unforeseen or unanticipated practical difficulties in following the intended research method. The pilot is very much like a dress rehearsal and is an indication of rigour. The flexible nature of qualitative research means that pilots are mainly a feature of quantitative than qualitative research, although a small practice interview or observation may be used in the latter.

Placebo effect: The power of suggestion in drug trials where the belief in the effectiveness of a drug can produce perceived positive outcomes reported by subjects. To reduce this, a non-active drug or treatment is used to act as a measure against the drug or procedure being tested and concealment as to who has the active drug is applied to as many in the setting as possible, including clinical staff.

Population: A clearly defined group who share common characteristics as specified by the researcher. The target population indicates those the researcher wants to say something about and the study population is the members of those groups that can be accessed to take part in the study.

Power analysis: Statistical procedure to calculate the size of a sample needed in a randomised control trial to ensure that the statistical calculations are sensitive and accurate.

Primary sources: A review of the literature in which the researcher consults the original authors and studies, and does not depend on secondary sources, which are summaries or descriptions by other authors of someone's work.

Probability sampling methods: A collection of strategies for selecting a sample from a population that results in a highly representative group. Strategies include simple random sampling, stratified sampling, proportionate sampling and cluster sampling methods. A number of sophisticated statistical techniques can be used on such samples.

Probing: In interviewing, a way of gaining more in-depth data by asking further questions to elaborate on points. This is not the same as prompting, where the interviewer offers a possible answer accepted by the respondent, although it may be inaccurate.

Proportionate random sampling: A method of ensuring that important subgroups in the sample are in the same proportions as those in the main population. This reduces the risk of bias through unevenly sized subgroups that might make a difference to the overall results.

Prospective study: A study where the data lies in the future at the start of the research. Newly occurring data are then collected as the study progresses. The opposite is a retrospective study, where the data already exist when the study is set up. Prospective studies have the advantage of greater control by the researcher, and therefore greater accuracy.

Purposive sampling: Also called judgemental sampling. This sampling strategy hand picks items or people on the basis of the researcher's prior knowledge of typical characteristics in the group. Despite sounding as though there is an element of bias here, this type of sample can produce a typical or representative sample.

Qualitative research: Broad heading for a number of research designs that are not so much concerned with numerical accuracy and the need to control or predict, but rather the need for insight and understanding. The findings are in the form of words and descriptions rather than numbers.

Quantitative research: Broad heading for a number of research designs to data gathering that produce numeric results. The concerns of this type of research centre on accuracy, the ability to generalise and to control and predict situations.

Quasi-experimental design: Used when random allocation may not be possible. This looks like an experimental study in that the researcher introduces an independent variable, but it uses groups that have not been randomly allocated. This means that the outcome might be due to factors other than the independent variable.

Questionnaire: Popular method of collecting research data that consists of respondents writing answers to a written set of questions and returning this to the researcher.

Quota sampling: A non-probability sampling strategy often used by market researchers where the researcher predetermines how many in the sample they will recruit with certain characteristics such as age or social class grouping. Once a particular quota is complete, emphasis is placed on the remaining categories.

Random allocation or Randomisation: The method of allocating those in a trial to the experimental or control group so that everyone has an equal chance of ending up in either group. Usually involves computer generated random numbers, tables of random numbers and sampling frames (lists of those eligible for allocation). Other techniques, such as picking names out of a hat or using the last digits on a medical record, are less well accepted as achieving a high level of randomisation.

Random selection: This ensures that everyone in a target population has an equal chance of being selected for study. Where data are gathered from everyone selected, the findings should be highly accurate and representative of the population as a whole. A number of statistical tests assume data are taken from such a random selection of the population.

Reactivity: A change in behaviour due to the taking part in a study and not related to anything introduced by the research. This distortion has an adverse effect on results.

Reliability: The accuracy of the tool of data collection. This is usually subject to a number of tests to ensure consistency. A pilot study will also be used to examine the reliability of the tool of data collection unless a well-used tool is applied.

Replication study: A design based on a study that has previously been carried out to confirm the findings of the first. Can take a number of different forms, including replication of the sampling design, the tool of data collection and other testing procedures.

Research: Extending knowledge and understanding through the systematic collection of information that answers a specific question objectively and as accurately as possible.

Research governance: Framework of accountability to be met by organisations within which research is carried out. The purpose is to ensure high standards of research through meeting ethical, scientific and safety criteria in the conduct of research. Additional accountability includes ensuring that the results of studies are communicated and accessible to those who can benefit from them.

Research proposal: An outline of an intended piece of research. It is used to gain ethical approval, permission or funding. It also allows the researcher to think through the whole process and identify any weak areas.

Research question: Related to the aim of a study, this is the element that structures the research process, particularly data collection, as the results of a study should answer this question.

Respect for persons: Part of the ethical code that relates to ensuring individuals are treated as autonomous, e.g. must be given the freedom to determine whether or not to participate in research.

Respondent: Term describing someone taking part in a study, often used in relation to questionnaires and interviews.

Response rate: The number of those returning a questionnaire or agreeing to be interviewed, expressed as a proportion of the total sent out or approached.

Results: Usually applied to the numeric findings of a study produced by data collection.

Retrospective study: A study in which the data already exist when the study is set up. These data cannot be influenced by the researcher, which reduces bias. The disadvantage is the lack of control over the quality of the data. The opposite of a prospective study.

Review of the literature: See *Literature review*.

Rigour: The extent to which the researcher has actively sought to carry out the study to a high standard. This includes identifying possible pitfalls in the design of the study and reducing their effect as much as possible. The end result should be a study that is as accurate and professional as possible.

Risk versus benefit ratio: Ethical principle of assessing whether the risks inherent in the study design are outweighed by possible benefits. These should be made known to those invited to take part in a study, particularly where the risks are high or of an unknown magnitude.

Sample: A section of a defined population used in a study to provide data.

Sampling frame: A list of all those who are eligible to be included in a study according to the inclusion/exclusion criteria. Each 'unit' in the list is numbered and, using a table of random numbers or computer generated random numbers, the researcher draws a predetermined set of numbers that are then matched against those in the sampling frame to provide the names or identity of those randomly selected.

Sample mortality: In experimental designs or longitudinal survey designs, e.g. cohort studies. This refers to participants who, for one reason or another (not necessarily death), leave the study. If there is a high mortality rate in one or more of the groups in an experimental design, those remaining in a study may no longer produce a typical group, making comparisons between groups unreliable.

Sampling strategy: Also referred to as a sampling plan. The choice of method used to select a sample for data collection.

Saturation: Also referred to as '*data saturation*'. In qualitative research, the point at which no new analytical categories or themes are arising from the data analysis, so the researcher ends data collection, as further data would be redundant.

Scientific approach: This is an ordered and objective method of collecting information in such a way as to provide verifiable data. Developed from the natural sciences, such as physics and chemistry, this approach has now been applied to human behaviour on the assumption that we are subject to similar constant patterns and influences. Those who favour a more humanistic approach, such as that of qualitative research, dispute this.

Secondary source: In reviewing the literature, where an author's original work is not consulted, only the work as cited, or outlined, by another author. There are dangers with this, as the primary source could be misquoted, or vital information omitted. The opposite of a primary source.

Selection bias: Where the sampling strategy used has not resulted in a representative group.

Self-report: Method of data collection that consists of asking people to provide information about themselves, such as in questionnaires, interviews or diaries. Built on the assumption that what people say they do is accurate, which might not always be the case.

Seminal study: Description of a study that was the first to tackle a topic and has become a 'classic'. It provided the 'seed' from which other studies have grown.

Semi-structured interview: A feature of qualitative interviews that contains some questions that are asked of everyone to ensure areas or topics of importance to the study are included; the remaining questions are more spontaneous and depend on the flow of conversation.

Simple random sample: A sampling strategy where everyone or every item has an equal chance of being selected. Requires a sampling frame and a table of random numbers or computer generated random numbers.

Snowball sampling: Also known as 'chain', 'nominated' or 'network' sampling. A sampling strategy used in qualitative research when it is difficult to identify or locate suitable candidates for the study. The procedure depends on finding some appropriate members, and then asking them for the names of contacts who might be willing to take part. The disadvantage is that, as the nominated people will be socially close to the individual, the resultant sample may not be representative of the wider group.

Social desirability: Found in surveys when individuals answer inaccurately because they want to be seen in a good light and give socially approved responses.

Stability: Refers to a tool of data collection that is consistent in its ability to provide accurate measurements.

Standard deviation: In statistics, an indication of the spread of values around the mean.

Stratified random sampling: Method of dividing the sampling frame into appropriate subgroups and drawing the sample from within each one.

Statistical significance: The extent to which the results of a study could have happened by chance rather than the result of an intervention or independent variable. This is indicated by the 'p' value.

Structured interview: Type of interview that has a high degree of structure. Basically, the researcher reads from a questionnaire (called an interview schedule) and writes down the answers. The advantage is that people may be more willing to engage in this as opposed to finding time to completing and returning a questionnaire. It also makes the answers more easily comparable with the minimum of coding. The disadvantage is respondents can only follow the line of questioning and wording laid down in the schedule.

Structured observation: The use of a list of behaviours that will focus the observer's attention. This usually results in a quantitative analysis of the frequency with which events occurred.

Subject: Used to refer to someone in a study. Has overtones of 'using' and seeing people as objects.

Survey: A research design that uses mainly questionnaires or interviews to collect descriptive data from a reasonably large sample.

Systematic sampling: Method of numbering all possible units in a sampling frame and then choosing units at a set interval, such as every tenth, to ensure that the entire range of the sample is included.

t-test: Statistical test that compares the means of two groups to establish if any differences between them could have happened by chance.

Theory: In quantitative research, the set of ideas about a situation that guides the construction of a study and its analysis. Hypotheses are developed from theories. In qualitative research using grounded theory, the findings may be used to construct a theory to explain them.

Thick data: In qualitative research, where the researcher has provided a great deal of descriptive detail to allow readers to feel as though they are there, or that will allow them to relate to what is going on.

Threats to internal or external validity: Factors that can provide an alternative explanation for the results of the study due to influences within the study (internal threats) or which reduce the ability to apply the results more widely (external threats).

Transferability: Also called fittingness. In qualitative research, the likelihood that the findings could provide insights into other situations.

Trend survey: This type of longitudinal study examines different groups of people from the same population at different times to identify any changes in the variable under study. This can include attitudes and experiences as well as physical, psychological or social changes. Following the same group over time would provide a '*panel*' study.

Triangulation: The use of more than one method of data collection in the same study in an attempt to produce more accurate information or understanding.

Trustworthiness: In qualitative research, one of the criteria used in establishing the authenticity and accuracy of the information presented. Can be compared to the concepts of reliability and validity in quantitative research.

Two-tailed hypothesis: Also called a non-directional hypothesis, this predicts a difference between two groups in the study but does not indicate in which direction. It simply states there will be a difference.

Unstructured interview: Also called a non-standardised interview. In qualitative research, used as a way of gaining an insight into a situation from the other person's or insider's perspective (emic view) without enforcing the researcher's point of view on the situation. Broad questions and probing are used where necessary to maintain the flow of ideas.

Unstructured observation: An in-depth form of observation used in qualitative research, such as ethnographic studies, where the researcher tries to record as much of what is happening as possible.

Variable: The item or 'thing' that forms the focus of the researcher's attention. Called a variable because such items vary in some way, e.g. temperature, pulse, age, gender, satisfaction with care, length of labour.

Validity: The extent to which a tool of data collection has produced what it was intended to produce.

Vignette: Used in questionnaires or interviews. Takes the form of a story, pen portrait or scenario on which the respondents answer questions to reveal their attitude, knowledge or behaviour. The problem is knowing if such answers really predict what a person would do in the actual situation.

Visual Analogue Scale (VAS): Measuring instrument in the form of a straight line. Respondents indicate their location between the two points on the line, e.g. Most pain ever felt/No pain, extreme anxiety/No anxiety. The points on the scale are given numerical values to allow for statistical analysis.

Vulnerable subjects: In ethical considerations, those people who are especially at risk and may not be in a position to give true informed consent, e.g. women in painful labour asked to provide consent to a procedure to which they would not agree in normal circumstances. Other vulnerable groups include children, those who are distressed, those with a challenged mental capacity, those with language difficulties and the unconscious.

INDEX

Note: Page numbers followed by *b* indicate boxes; *f* figures; *t* tables.

A
Accidental sampling, surveys, 206–207
Action research design, 35
Advocacy, ethics, 102–103
Agreement scales, questionnaire design, 125
Allocation concealment, 159–160
Analysis, inductive, 47
Anonymity, informed consent, 109
Attention factor, 158
Audit, 220
  definition, 17–18
  research *vs.*, 17
Auditability
  qualitative research, 58
Audit trails, data analysis, 73–74
Autonomy, ethics, 107–109
Avoiding harm, ethics, 109–110

B
Back chaining, literature sourcing, 82
Bar charts, 184*t*, 187–188
Barriers to research, 217–218
Basic human rights, 106–111
The Belmont report, 103
Beneficence, 4, 109–110
Bias, 26, 29
  experiments, 168
  observer, 150
  questionnaire design, 124
  randomisation effects, 158
Binomial distribution, 181
Blinding, experiments, 159–160
Bracketing, phenomenology, 51

C
Categorical level, descriptive statistics, 176–177, 178*t*
Central tendency measures, descriptive statistics, 178–179
Chain sampling, qualitative research, 208–209
Checklists, observation, 147
Chi-squared test (χ^2), 192*t*
Closed questions, questionnaires, 124–125
Closing of interviews, 139
Cluster sampling, surveys, 205
Cochrane Collaboration database, 34

Cohort study, 118–119
Complex hypotheses, 97–98
Concept definitions, 23–24, 28
  experiments, 170
  structured observation, 144–145
Conceptual frameworks (maps), 24–25, 25*f*, 29
Conceptual phase of research, 31
Confidence intervals (CI), 188
Confidentiality, 111
  informed consent, 109
  interviews, 140
Confirmability, trustworthiness, 73
Consent, informed *see* Informed consent
Constant comparison method, data analysis, 52
Constructivist research *see* Qualitative research
Contingency table, 185
Control, experiments, 159–160, 169
Convenience sampling
  qualitative research, 208
  surveys, 206–207
Correlation coefficient, 189–190
Correlations, 189–191
  calculation, 190–191, 190*f*
  direction of, 189
  multiple regression, 191
  strength of, 189
Correlation, strength of, 189
Credibility
  qualitative research, 58
  trustworthiness, 72
Critiquing research, 13–14, 27–28, 40–41, 223–224
  ethics, 113
  experiments, 169–170
  interviews, 141
  literature reviews, 88
  observation, 151–152
  qualitative research, 57–58
  research questions, 98–99
  sample size, 212
  sampling methods, 211–212
  statistics, 194–195
  surveys, 129
Cross-sectional survey, 118
Cross-tabulation table, 185
Cultural strangeness
  ethnography, 49–50
  observation, 149

243

D

Data
  security, 109
  statistics, 174
  summation, 193
  type, study planning, 36
Data analysis, 39
  grounded theory, 52
  qualitative research, 73–74
  research approach, 131–132
  study planning, 37
  see also Statistics
Databases, literature sourcing, 81
Data collection, 38–39
  qualitative research, 19, 46–47, 72
  study planning, 36–37
  see also specific methods
Data presentation
  qualitative research, 19
  quantitative research, 19
Data saturation, qualitative research, 73
The declaration of Helsinki, 103
Declarative research questions, 94
Demographic data, surveys, 119
Dependability
  data analysis, 73–74
  trustworthiness, 73
Dependent variables, 22, 23t
  experiments, 170
Descriptive approach, level 1 questions, 21
Descriptive statistics, 174–176
  bar charts, 184t, 187–188
  central tendency measures, 178–179
  histograms, 184t, 187
  interval level, 177, 178t
  levels of measurement, 176–179, 178t
    see also specific levels
  line graphs, 184t
  mean, 179–188
  median, 180–181
  mode, 181–182
  nominal (categorical) level, 176–177, 178t
  normal distributions, 182–184, 183f
  ordinal level, 177, 178t
  pie charts, 184t, 187–188
  ratio level, 177–178, 178t
  result presentation, 184–188, 184t
    see also specific methods
  standard distributions, 182
  tables, 184t, 185–186
Design and planning phase of research, 31
Directional hypotheses, 96
Direction of correlation, 189
Dissemination phase of research, 31
Drift, observer, 150

E

Eligibility criteria, 198
Empirical phase of research, 31
Ethics, 101–115
  advocacy, 102–103
  avoiding harm, 109–110
  basic human rights, 106–111
  definition, 101
  evidence-based practice, 4
  experiments, 168, 169

Ethics *(Continued)*
  historical development, 104
  individual autonomy, 107–109
  international codes, 103b
  justice, 110–111
  observation, 148
  researchers, 102
  research governance, 104–105
  subjects of research, 102
Ethnography, 47, 49–50, 58–59
  'cultural strangeness', 49–50
  definition, 49
  fieldwork, 49–50
  'going native', 49–50
  observation, 151
  unstructured observation, 146
Evaluation scales, questionnaire design, 125
Evidence-based practice, 1–15
  definition, 3
  developments in, 5–7
  ethics, 4
  increase in, 5
  PICO (Population–Intervention–Comparison–Outcome), 7
  process of, 7–9, 8f
  reasons for, 4
  research *vs.*, 3–4
Evidence, source comparison, 11–13, 12t
Exclusion criteria, 26, 198–199
Experiment(s), 155–171
  bias, 168
  blinding, 159–160
  concept definitions, 170
  control, 159–160, 169
  dependent variables, 170
  ethics, 168, 169
  ex post facto studies, 167
  hypothesis, 160–161, 168
  importance of, 155–156
  independent variables, 170
  information needed, 168
  level 3 questions, 21
  manipulation, 158–159, 169
  operational definitions, 170
  planning, 167
  post-test only design, 162–163, 163f
  pre-test post-test control group, 162, 162f
  quasi-experimental design, 166
  randomisation, 157–158, 169
  sampling, 200t
  sampling methods, 199–203
  Solomon four-group design, 163, 163f
  types, 161–163
  validity threats, 164–166
Experimental design, 156–160
  multifactorial influences, 22–23
  sample size, 209–210
Ex post facto studies, 167
  sampling, 200t, 203–204
External validity, experiments, 165

F

Feminist research, 54–56, 59
  definition, 55
Fieldwork
  ethnography, 49–50
  qualitative research, 47

Fieldwork diary
  grounded theory, 52
  qualitative research, 74
Findings, communication of *see* Result presentation
Fittingness, qualitative research, 58
Focus groups, 137–138
  disadvantages, 137
  moderators, 137
  size, 137
  skills needed, 139
Forward chaining, literature sourcing, 82
Frequency distribution, structured observation, 144
Frequency scales, questionnaire design, 125
Frequency tables, 185

G

Going native
  ethnography, 49–50
  observation, 149
Grand tour questions, 132
Grey literature, 78
Grounded theory, 47, 51–52, 58–59

H

Harm avoidance, ethics, 109–110
Hawthorne effect, 158
Heidegger, Martin, 51
Histograms, 184*t*, 187
Historic research, research design, 35
Homogeneity of variance, 189
Human rights, 106–111
Husserl, Edmund, 51
Hypotheses, 32–33, 95–98, 160–161
  complex, 97–98
  definition, 95
  directional (one-tailed), 96
  experiments, 160–161, 168
  non-directional (two-tailed), 96–97
  null *see* Null hypotheses
  one-tailed, 168
  purpose, 96
  research *see* Research hypotheses
  scientific *see* Research hypotheses
  two-tailed, 168
  see also specific types

I

Inclusion criteria, 26
  sampling methods, 198–199
Independent *t*-test, 192*t*
Independent variables, 22, 23*t*
  experiments, 170
Individual autonomy, ethics, 107–109
Inductive analysis, 47
Inferential statistics, 188–192
  confidence intervals (CI), 188
  correlation *see* Correlation
  hypothesis support, 188
  non-parametric tests, 189
  parametric tests, 189
  probability estimation, 188
  tests of significance, 191–192, 192*t*
  see also specific tests

Informed consent, 108, 111
  anonymity, 109
  confidentiality, 109
  information, 108, 108*b*
  language used, 108
  written consent, 109
Instrumentation, internal experimental validity, 164
Integrated literature reviews, 77
Intellectual property, research governance, 105–106
Interactive effects, internal experimental validity, 165
Internal validity, experiments, 164
International codes, ethics, 103*b*
International Review Boards (IRBs), 106
  see also Local Research Ethics Committees (LRECs)
Inter-rate reliability, 159
Interrogative research questions, 94
Interval level, descriptive statistics, 177, 178*t*
Interview(s), 131–142
  advantages, 131–132, 133–134, 133*b*
  answer recording, 135–136
  closing of, 139
  confidentiality, 140
  definition, 131–132
  disadvantages, 133–134, 134*b*
  environment, 135
  focus groups *see* Focus groups
  free-flowing, 140
  grand tour questions, 132
  grounded theory, 52
  with health professionals, 139–140
  interviewer influence, 133–134
  interviewer's appearance, 135
  principles, 134–136
  result presentation, 141
  role-play, 134–135
  semi-structured, 132–133
  skills needed, 133, 138–139
  socially desirable answers, 133–134
  structure, 132–133, 140
  telephone *see* Telephone interviews
  unstructured (non-standardized), 132
  women-centred approach, 133
Interview guides, 132
Interview schedule, 132

J

Jargon/nomenclature, 18
Justice, ethics, 110–111

K

Key words
  literature reviews, 79, 79*b*
  literature sourcing, 81

L

Level 1 research questions, 20–21, 20*t*, 93, 94*t*
Level 2 research questions, 20*t*, 21, 93, 94*t*
Level 3 research questions, 20*t*, 21, 93, 94*t*
Levels of measurement, descriptive statistics, 176–179, 178*t*
Likert scales, questionnaire design, 126
Line graphs, 184*t*

Literature reviews, 10, 34, 77–89, 223
  common questions, 85
  definition, 77
  detail extraction, 83
  grey literature, 78
  integrated, 77
  key words, 79, 79b
  meta-analysis, 77
  meta-synthesis (meta-studies), 78
  narrative, 77
  planning, 79, 80b
  processes, 79–80, 79b
  qualitative research, 34
  reasons for, 78
  sourcing *see* Literature sourcing
  systemic reviews, 77
  writing of, 85–86
  see also Critiquing research articles
Literature sourcing, 80–82
  back chaining, 82
  databases, 81
  forward chaining, 82
  journal articles, 80
  key words, 81
  questions needed, 81
  search engines, 81–82
Local Research Ethics Committees (LRECs), 102, 104–105, 106, 112
Logical reasoning, 12t
Longitudinal survey, 118–119
LRECs *see* Local Research Ethics Committees (LRECs)

M

Manipulation, experiments, 158–159, 169
Mann–Whitney *U* test, 192t
Maturation, internal experimental validity, 164
Mean, 179–188
Measurement effects, experimental validity, 165
Measurement levels, descriptive statistics, 176–179
Median, 180–181
Member's check, trustworthiness, 72
Merleau-Ponty, Maurice, 51
Meta-analysis, literature reviews, 77
Meta-studies, literature reviews, 78
Meta-synthesis, literature reviews, 78
Methodological issues
  definition, 17
  qualitative research, 72–73
MIDIRS (*Midwives Information and Resource Service*), 6–7, 34
Mode, 181–182
Moderators, focus groups, 137
Mortality, internal experimental validity, 164–165
Multimodal distribution, 181
Multiple regression, correlation, 191
Multistage sampling, 206

N

Negative case analysis, trustworthiness, 72
Network sampling, qualitative research, 208–209
Nominal level, descriptive statistics, 176–177, 178t

Nominated sampling, qualitative research, 208–209
Non-directional hypotheses, 96–97
Non-equivalent control group design, 166
Non-maleficence, 4, 109–110
Non-parametric tests, inferential statistics, 189
Non-standardized interviews, 132
Non-verbal skills, interviews, 138
Normal distributions, 182–184, 183f
Null hypotheses, 97, 160–161, 168
  example, 161b
The Nuremberg code, 103
Nursing guidelines, ethics, 104

O

Observation, 143–153
  advantages, 147–148
  definition, 143–144
  disadvantages, 148–150
  grounded theory, 52
  reasons for, 144
  recording, 147
  structured, 143, 144–145
  unstructured, 143, 145–147
Observer bias, 150
Observer drift, 150
Observer fatigue, 150
Observer roles, 145–146, 146b
One-tailed hypotheses, 96
On-line surveys, 127
Open questions, questionnaires, 124–125
Operational definitions, 23–24, 28
  experiments, 170
Opportunity sampling, surveys, 206–207
Ordinal level, descriptive statistics, 177, 178t

P

Panel survey, 118–119
Paradigms, 43
Parametric tests, 189
Patient-related outcome measures (PROMs), 219
Pearson correlation, 192t
Pearson product moment, 190–191
Peer reviewed articles, 81–82
Phenomenology, 47, 50–51, 58–59
  bracketing, 51
  critiquing qualitative research, 69
  definition, 50–51
PICO (Population–Intervention–Comparison–Outcome), 7
Pie charts, 184t, 187–188
Pilot studies, 38
Popularity, surveys, 117–118
Population–Intervention–Comparison–Outcome (PICO), 7
Populations, samples *vs.*, 197
Post-test only design, 162–163, 163f
Power analysis, sample size, 209–210
Pre-test post-test control group, 162, 162f
Probability estimation, inferential statistics, 188
Probability methods, sampling methods, 199–200
Probability values, 155–156, 156b
PROMs (patient-related outcome measures), 219

Proportionate sampling, 203
   surveys, 205
Purposive sampling, qualitative research, 208

Q

Qualitative research, 18–20, 28, 43–60
   aim, 71–72
   application to clinical practise, 74
   background, 71–72
   chain sampling, 208–209
   characteristics, 45*b*
   conclusions, 74
   convenience sampling, 208
   data analysis, 47, 73–74
   data collection, 19, 46–47
   data interpretation, 47
   data presentation, 19
   data saturation, 73
   definition, 19, 44, 58
   design, 47–52
      see also Ethnography; Grounded theory; Phenomenology
   ethics, 56, 57, 73
   feminist research *see* Feminist research
   fieldwork diary, 74
   methodological issues, 72–73
   network sampling, 208–209
   nominated sampling, 208–209
   observation, 147, 148
   planning, 45–46
   purposive sampling, 208
   quantitative research *vs.*, 27, 43, 44–47, 48*t*
   questions, 56
   researcher–sample relationship, 46, 57
   sample size, 73, 210–211
   sampling, 200*t*, 207–209
      see also specific methods
   snowball sampling, 208–209
   theoretical sampling, 209
Quantitative research, 18–20, 28
   data presentation, 19
   definition, 18
   qualitative research *vs.*, 27, 43, 44–47, 48*t*
   telephone interviews, 136
Quasi-experimental, sampling, 200*t*, 203–204
Question choice, questionnaires, 122–123, 128
Questionnaires, 119–121
   advantages, 120*b*
   answer design, 124–127
   closed questions, 124–125
   design, 121–124, 123*b*
   disadvantages, 120*b*
   instructions, 122
   length, 122–123
   open questions, 124–125
   participation invitation, 121, 122*b*
   question choice, 122–123, 128
   response analysis, 126–127
   return of, 127
   self-completing, 119
   structure, 123–124
   unanswered questions, 120–121
   wording, 123–124
Questions
   see also Research questions
Quota sampling, surveys, 207–209

R

Random allocation, 157–158, 200–201
Random assignment, 157–158
Randomisation, experiments, 157–158, 169
Randomised control trials (RCTs), 155, 219
Random numbers, 201–202, 201*b*
Random samples/sampling, 199–200
   random numbers, 201–202, 201*b*
   sampling frames, 201
   study population, 201
Ratio level, descriptive statistics, 177–178, 178*t*
RCTs *see* Randomised control trials (RCTs)
Reactive effects, experimental validity, 165
Reactivity, observation, 148, 149
Recording
   observation, 147
   structured observation, 145
Reflective journals, trustworthiness, 72
Reflexivity, data collection, 47
Regression, internal experimental validity, 164
Reliability, 25–26, 29
Research, 12*t*
   accessibility, 3
   accuracy, 10
   audit *vs.*, 17
   availability, 3
   barriers to, 217–218
   culture development, 220–221
   definition, 17
   disadvantages, 13
   as evidence, 9–11
   evidence-based practice *vs.*, 3–4
   evidence collection, 10
   framework of, 31–41, 32*b*
   key concepts, 17–29
      see also specific concepts
   production *vs.* use of, 216–217
   see also Experiment(s); *specific types*
Research aims, research questions, 95, 95*t*
Research Ethics Committee (REC), 40
Research governance, 104–106
   ethics, 104–105
   finance, 105–106
   health, safety and environment, 105
   information, 105
   intellectual property, 105–106
   science, 105
Research hypotheses, 97, 160–161
Research proposals
   ethics, 112
   sampling methods, 198–199
Research questions, 20–21, 20*t*, 28, 32–33, 33*t*, 91–100
   construction of, 94–95
   data collection methods, 93–94
   declarative, 94
   feasibility, 33, 92
   interrogative, 94
   level 1, 20–21, 20*t*, 93, 94*t*
   level 2, 20*t*, 21, 93, 94*t*
   level 3, 20*t*, 21, 93, 94*t*
   level identification, 27
   qualitative research, 56
   research aims, 95, 95*t*
   role of, 91–93
   types of, 93–94, 94*t*
      see also specific types
   see also Hypotheses

Response analysis, questionnaires, 126–127
Response discouragement, questionnaires, 120
Result presentation, 39–40, 222
 descriptive statistics, 184–188, 184t
 interviews, 141
Retrospective studies, 167
Reviews, literature see Literature reviews
Ricoeur, Paul, 51
Rigour, 26–27, 29
 study planning, 34–35

S

Sample(s)
 populations vs., 197
 representativeness, surveys, 119
 study planning, 36
Sample attrition, 210
Sample mortality, 210
Sample size, 209–211
 experimental design, 209–210
 power analysis, 209–210
 qualitative research, 73, 210–211
 surveys, 210
Sampling
 experiments, 200t
 ex post facto studies, 200t, 203–204
 intervals, 205
 multistage, 206
 qualitative research, 200t, 207–209
 quasi-experimental, 200t, 203–204
 surveys, 200t, 204–207, 211
Sampling bias, 198
Sampling frames, random sampling, 201
Sampling methods, 197–213
 exclusion criteria, 198–199
 experimental approaches, 199–203
 inclusion criteria, 198–199
 probability methods, 199–200
 proportionate sampling, 203
 random methods, 199–200
 reasons for, 198
 research proposals, 198–199
 sampling bias, 198
 simple random sample, 200–202
 stratified samples, 202–203
 see also specific methods
Scaling techniques, questionnaire design, 125
Scientific hypotheses see Research hypotheses
Search engines, literature sourcing, 81–82
Selection effects, experimental validity, 165
Selectivity, observation, 149–150
Self-completing, questionnaires, 119
Semi-structured interviews, 132–133
Significance
 statistics, 174
 tests of, 191–192, 192t
Simple random sampling, 200–202
 surveys, 204
Snowball sampling, 208–209
Socially desirable answers, interviews, 133–134
Solomon four-group experimental design, 163, 163f
Spearman's coefficient, 192t
Spearman's rho, 190–191, 192t
Standard distributions, 182

Statistics, 173–195
 common symbols, 175t
 data, 174
 data input, 193
 descriptive see Descriptive statistics
 experiments, 169, 170
 inferential see Inferential statistics
 significance, 174
Stratified sampling, 202–203
 surveys, 204
Strength of correlation, 189
Structured observation, 143, 144–145
Student's t-test, 192t
Study mortality, surveys, 118–119
Study population, random sampling, 201
Subject mortality, Solomon four-group experimental design, 163
Surveys, 117–130
 cohort study, 118–119
 cross-sectional survey, 118
 definition, 117
 demographic data, 119
 disadvantages, 118
 longitudinal survey, 118–119
 on-line, 127
 panel survey, 118–119
 questionnaires see Questionnaires
 sampling see below
 structure, 118
 study mortality, 118–119
 trend survey, 118
 types, 118
 validity, 119
Surveys, sampling, 200t, 204–207, 211
 accidental sampling, 206–207
 cluster sampling, 205
 convenience sampling, 206–207
 opportunity sampling, 206–207
 proportionate sampling, 205
 quota sampling, 207–209
 sample representativeness, 119
 sample size, 210
 simple random sampling, 204
 stratified sampling, 204
 systemic sampling, 205
Symbols, statistics, 175t
Systemic reviews, literature reviews, 77
Systemic sampling, surveys, 205

T

Tables, 184t, 185–186
 randomised control trials (RCTs), 187
Telephone interviews, 136–137
 advantages, 136–137
 disadvantages, 137
 length of, 137
 quantitative design, 136
Term of reference, questions, 32
Testing, internal experimental validity, 164
Tests of significance, 191–192, 192t
Theoretical frameworks, 24–25, 29
Theoretical sampling, qualitative research, 209
Transferability, trustworthiness, 73
Trend survey, 118
Trial and error, 12t
Triangulation, data collection, 46
Trustworthiness, qualitative research, 72

T-test, 192t
Two-tailed hypotheses, 96–97

U
Unrelated experimental groups, 162
Unstructured interviews, 132
Unstructured observation, 143, 145–147

V
Validity, 26, 29
 surveys, 119
 threats, experiments, 164–166
Variables, 22–23, 23t, 28
 dependent *see* Dependent variables
 identification, 27–28
 independent *see* Independent variables

Variance, homogeneity of, 189
Visual analog scales (VAS), 24
 questionnaire design, 126

W
Wilcoxon test, 192t
Women-centred approach,
 interviews, 133
Women-related outcome measures
 (WROMs), 219
Wording, questionnaires,
 123–124
Writing
 literature reviews, 85–86
Written consent, 109
WROMs (women-related outcome
 measures), 219